PROPHETS & PRIESTS

The Hidden Face
of the Birth Control Movement

To the Hancocks and the Maidments, my grandparents, who according to the Birth Controllers should certainly never have been allowed to 'breed'. To my dear Father, who actually experienced the results of Malthus's plan to control the numbers of the poor by separating the sexes in the Workhouse.

May they rest in peace.

PROPHETS & PRIESTS

The Hidden Face
of the Birth Control Movement

Ann Farmer

The Saint Austin Press
296, Brockley Road, London, SE4 2RA
MMII

THE SAINT AUSTIN PRESS
296, Brockley Road
London, SE4 2RA

Telephone: +44 (0)20 8692 6009
Facsimile: +44 (0)20 8469 3609

Electronic mail: books@saintaustin.org
http://www.saintaustin.org

ISBN 1 901157 62 8
Copyright © Ann Farmer, 2002.

Printed by Newton Printing Ltd, London, U.K. www.newtonprinting.com

TABLE OF CONTENTS

FOREWORD

In his seminal work on the history of sexuality, the French philosopher Michel Foucault commented on the intention of some to administer and control the fertility of others, which arose at the end of the nineteenth century. He described the resulting programme of eugenics (I believe with some irony) as one of the '... great innovations in the technology of sex of the second half of the nineteenth century.' (1) One of the new, discursive 'types' of subjects created from these times included the Malthusian Couple, good citizens who would faithfully, in their very thoughts as well as their actions, actively submit to the requirements of the burgeoning eugenic doctrine.

The Malthusian couple as a discursive 'type' survives to this very day. This stereotype arose initially from bourgeois preoccupations and anxieties about the 'lower' classes and their children. Ann Farmer's groundbreaking account of these preoccupations, from the nineteenth century to much more recent history, examines the underlying motives of the eugenicists and would-be birth controllers expressed in their own words. In doing so, she is likely to cause discomfiture to many. For the prejudices, obsessions and indifference to suffering that such prominent figures exhibited have often been hidden from public knowledge by previous authors: where birth control had come to be seen as a social benefit in the latter part of the twentieth century, by libertarians and feminists alike, the continuing legacy of its dark beginnings was pragmatically and persistently suppressed or ignored. This book is, in some ways, an uncomfortable read; various historical figures previously hailed as heroes of sexual freedom and personal liberty are revealed to have been motivated primarily by sinister leanings. For modern feminists, especially, who have often subscribed to the idea that such movers and shakers in the birth control movement were feminist heroines and heroes, this account may be particularly difficult to read.

Yet read it they must. A thorough critical engagement with the history of the eugenics and birth control movements in Britain, in all their guises, as revealed in their own words, is long overdue. The messy, complex and worrying effects of their intervention in so many people's lives also has needed to be documented, and this book fulfils that need too. The almost religious zeal of the secular eugenicists and birth-controllers to influence the members of the society in which they lived to adopt, uncritically and without question, a 'Malthusian' lifestyle, and its ramifications today, has given rise to the title of this book. Occasional claims to commitment to liberty for all belied their investment in the status, authority, power and privilege their claims to expertise entailed. In many important ways this work is one of a growing number of ongoing, rigorous interrogations, of the various Grand Narratives that have been made by privileged gentleman (and in later times, ladies), from the time of the Enlightenment to the present day. Only in such undertakings can we hope to learn from past (and present) mistakes to enable the possibility of a better future.

1. Foucault~ M. history of sexuality, volume 1: an introduction (1980) penguin, London, p 118.

Angela Kennedy, September 2001.

Angela Kennedy is a researcher at the Gender Research department at Middlesex University, where she gained a Master's degree in issues of gender and the body, and is now researching for a Doctorate in this field. She edited Swimming *Against the Tide: Feminist Dissent on the Issue of Abortion*, in 1997.

ACKNOWLEDGEMENTS

The author wishes to acknowledge the support and assistance received in the preparation of this work, in particular to Angela Kennedy for her feminist insights and unfailing support of the aims of the book. To my son Christopher and husband Alan for their technical support, and the following who have helped in the 'birth' of *Prophets and Priests*: Professor Jack Scarisbrick, Dr Helen Watt, Lord David Alton, Bishop Ambrose Griffiths, Kerry Pollard, MP, Kevin McNamara, MP, Bishop Thomas McMahon, Joanna Bogle, Sir Patrick Duffy, Bishop Christopher Budd, Cardinal Cormac Murphy-O-Connor, Dr Andrew Fergusson, Tom Mahon, the Bishop of Shrewsbury, Fr. Noel Barber, Bob O'Donnell and the Labour Life Group, the Bishop of East Anglia, Angela Appleby, Ferdi McDermott and the many others who contributed their good wishes and support.

INTRODUCTION

Everyone knows the story of the birth control campaign. It was a war fought by feminists and radicals against ignorance, superstition and the subjugation of women by Church and State,[1] a war that, by the beginning of the twenty-first century, has been largely won - in the developed world, if not in the poorer countries. It has been celebrated as a victory for sex equality, alongside successes like equal pay and votes for women.

Birth control is seen (variously) as the prerequisite of women's freedom and equality; integral to women's health; necessary for the well being of families; essential for the prosperity of the nation; urgently needed for the stability of the world; vital for the future of the planet. Everyone, it seems, agrees that birth control is a good thing. Among the 'great and the good' in science, medicine and politics, there are very few dissenters. Radicals and conservatives, men and women, young and old, even the rich man in his castle, and the poor man at his gate, sing in harmony on this issue. In an amazing first, feminist rhetoric joins hands with boring suburban commonsense, and disappears into the sunset.

Some see birth control as a good thing, most, as a neutral issue. Some see it as a minor evil best left alone. Few campaign against it any more, and those who do, have little impact. In the view of the majority in respectable Western society, the issue is cut and dried. The time before birth control is seen as the Dark Ages. How on earth did people live without it?

While the overwhelming majority fails to see abortion as a good thing, birth control is considered a quite separate issue. They appear to have grown up as two historically distinct campaigns. Family planning workers, toiling cheerfully to break down the barriers of ignorance and superstition, are the familiar face of the birth control movement; and surely their work is vital in avoiding abortions?

The acceptance of birth control is now virtually complete. Histories of birth control show that dissent on the issue was invariably linked with right-wing politics. Past opponents of birth control have been portrayed in social histories as reactionary anti-feminists, happy for women to have large families and be chained to the kitchen sink, 'barefoot and pregnant'. They have even been dubbed 'racist', and their views linked with those of Hitler and Mussolini.[2] Today, anyone voicing doubts about birth control may be accused of helping to increase the number of abortions, by denying women the means of preventing unwanted pregnancies.

Occasionally, birth control disasters such as Pill scares, abortifacient methods being presented as contraception, and the use of coercion or bribery in Third World countries, give a distinct feeling of unease. Such stories are soon forgotten, however, as the trickle of news dries up, and more sensational stories take their place. And anyway, as we enter the twenty-first century, and human cloning becomes a reality, surely it is time to leave ancient controversies about birth control behind?

But we *are* still concerned with injustice, especially in far away places; and family planning in far away places has a habit of slipping into coercion. Birth control is seen as a good thing – but when birth control is enforced on others, it is called population control, which is seen as bad. There has been no shortage of critics of population control, and they have made a valuable contribution to the study of birth control history, and its abuses. But most have failed to identify the crucial part played in the population control story by the abortion issue.[3]

The use of abortion as an abuse of human rights receives little attention even from those most closely concerned with fighting human oppression. Disguising abortion as contraception is the commonest example of abuse, and it affects a great many women who use birth control;[4] however, when forced abortion and even infanticide in China and Tibet attracts scant protest from feminists and human rights advocates, we are forced to conclude that abortion is an issue above criticism, however oblique.

Birth control, population control and abortion are seen as three separate issues, developing from three distinct strands of history. However, there are links between the three, which clearly demonstrate that this perception is dangerously mistaken. So many disturbing features have been covered up, overlooked, or downplayed by historians, that it is time for those concerned with human rights – since birth control has been presented as a human right[5] – to ask why.

Once we start to look into the history of birth control, we find many warnings to proceed no further. These warnings have a salutary effect. They tell us that the opponents of birth control were Catholic, or right-wing, or both; that birth control has always been practised by women eager to control their fertility; that the well-known supporters of the birth control movement were 'distinguished' and 'eminent', while the lesser-known campaigners were 'fearless' and 'indomitable'. We find that the poor were hungry for knowledge about birth control, which however was withheld from them by a State fearful of unleashing the sexuality of the poor, and by a Church bent on the spiritual subjugation of the people, especially women. We discover that the opponents of birth control were a motley crowd of crackpots and prudes.

Fearing to be associated with religious zealots, we are reluctant to proceed further. Tentative enquiries reveal that the early birth control campaigners mention abortion frequently – but only to roundly condemn it. This is even more puzzling, and rather contradicts the portrait of birth control advocates as brave and fearless.

Abortion is somehow never absent from the picture. We find that since the beginning of the birth control campaign, abortion has featured as the tragic problem, and birth control as the solution. However, experience has taught that the failure of contraception often leads to abortion, and further study reveals that even the most ardent family planners have long admitted this to be the

2

case.[6] The fact that many of the founders of the abortion campaign also worked for birth control,[7] leads to the conclusion that perhaps the two issues are better studied together, so that a better understanding of their origins may be achieved. What is the truth behind this strange, symbiotic relationship?

The truth is that birth control was initially regarded by most of society with abhorrence. This fact has been downplayed by historians. However, most of these have had links with the birth control campaign.[8] The study of how birth control came to be accepted within a few generations as beneficial, despite dangers, drawbacks and disasters, is fascinating and instructive. It also shows that history is being repeated, and that eventually abortion will become as acceptable and indispensable a part of life as birth control is today. And if it does, surely we would be wrong to withhold it as a means of development assistance to the Third World?

For this reason alone, the study of birth control history cannot be seen as an irrelevance. It is essential for anyone concerned with human rights and human wrongs, whether or not they are religious, and whatever their views on birth control. *Prophets & Priests* does not explore the religious arguments for or against birth control, but springs from extensive investigations into the history of population control and eugenics. However, women's personal experience of birth control has, perhaps more than any other factor, influenced this work. Many people's day-to-day experiences have totally failed to agree with the positive picture found in the histories of the birth control movement. Some, indeed, have **paid** the price of experience with their lives.

Opinions on abortion and on birth control vary, among people of all religious faiths and none. The two issues are, of course, dramatically different,[9] though few would see abortion as a good thing *per se*. But whatever the views, it is difficult, if not impossible, to reach any final conclusion without knowing all the facts, and no conclusion can be reached when certain vital pieces are missing from the jigsaw. *Prophets & Priests* does not set out to direct the reader to any particular conclusion; it intends to put the missing pieces back in the puzzle. Above all, it tells a fascinating story, and as we stand on the brink of the next great adventure in reproductive technology – cloning – we would do well to study the history of the very first attempts at controlling human reproduction.

Religion does feature in the history of the birth control story. It has often been seen by birth controllers as an obstacle to their campaign. This should not be too surprising, since from the very beginning, the birth control movement itself had all the hallmarks of a religion – and one that did not tolerate rivals easily. It, too, had its prophets and priests, some of whom are famous, others less so. They share one thing in common, however: their true faces have, until now, been largely hidden from public view.

NOTES

[1] "Women did not lose control of fertility overnight. Women experienced a long and bloody struggle with the combined weight of Church and State." (*Abortion, Liberation and Revolution*, International Marxist Group, 1979, p3)

[2] "...the Nazis were held in some esteem by the League [of National Life]...which called attention to the heroic efforts of Hitler and Mussolini to increase the birth rates of the white races..." (Madeleine Simms, 'British Women and their Enemies', in 'Who are the Anti-Abortionists?' (pamphlet), National Abortion Campaign, 1979)

[3] See Linda Gordon, Woman's Body, Woman's Right; Germaine Greer, Sex and Destiny; Stephen Trombley, the Right to Reproduce.

[4] The IUD can work as a contraceptive or an abortifacient. (See Germaine Greer, *Sex and Destiny*, Pan Books Ltd, London, 1985) The progesterone-only contraceptive pill (the 'mini-pill'), and the combined progesterone-oestrogen pill do not always prevent ovulation, but can prevent a fertilized egg from implanting in the womb. (John Wilks, *A Consumer's Guide to the Pill and other Drugs*, TGB Books, Australia, 1996, ISBN 0 646 29226 9) In the case of the 'Morning After Pill', or 'Post-coital pill', efforts have been made to disguise its abortifacient effects by redefining conception as implantation, as in the following:

"As you mention in your letter, emergency contraception prevents a fertilised egg from implanting in the womb. Although I fully appreciate that your own personal views may differ, the medical and legal view is that a pregnancy begins at implantation in the endometrium, not when the egg is fertilised. Emergency treatment cannot disrupt an existing pregnancy where the egg has implanted and, therefore, is not considered to be abortion." (Personal communication from the Department of Health, 5.6.1995) Also:

"The Pill. How it works. Alters hormone balance. This usually prevents pregnancy.

"The IUD. How it works. Acts in the womb. This usually prevents pregnancy." ('Emergency Contraception', (leaflet), The Family Planning Information Service; supported jointly by the Family Planning Association and the Health Education Authority, (1990).

In the drive to get women to accept abortifacients, they have even been portrayed as a means of avoiding abortion: "Pill that saves: 180,000 women have abortions they don't need", (*Daily Express*, 25.11.94)

[5] 'The Human Right to Family Planning', (booklet), International Planned Parenthood Federation, November 1983.

[6] The early birth controllers Helena Wright and Stella Browne recognised that abortion was necessary because of contraceptive failure. (For a study of contraceptive failure leading to unplanned pregnancy, see Haroulla Filakti, *Trends in Abortion 1990-95*, in *Population Trends 87*, Spring 1997, pp11-19.) Modern abortion advocates, including Malcolm Potts and Suzanne Moore, also acknowledge the necessity. Some organisations have also begun to agree: "...the legitimacy of induced abortion as a necessary back-up to contraceptive failure." ('Five-Year Plan – 1976-1980', Planned Parenthood of America) "...abortion is the last resort when other safeguards fail." ('Free Safe Abortion in the Eighties', (leaflet), TUC South-East Regional Council, n.d.) The development of thought in the Family Planning Association is interesting. In April 1966, a FPA Conference debated whether abortion should be made legal and part of normal practice under the National Health Service. (Abortion Law Reform Association papers (SA/FPA); in 1968, the FPA supported the Pregnancy Advisory Service in their lobbying for the extension of abortion services; in 1970, the FPA, with ALRA, set up the Birth Control Campaign to lobby for abortion, sterilisation, contraception, and to alert the Government on population problems. (*Abortion and Eugenics*, Fr. John Berry); the FPA now dispenses 'morning-after' abortifacients: "Unprotected intercourse may be the result of failure to use contraception or due to a method failure, such as a burst sheath." ('Postcoital Contraception', FPA Fact Sheet C7, (March 1983)) Even the World Health Organisation now recognises the significance of contraceptive failure leading to abortion, as the following shows: "The imperfections of currently available methods of

contraception were highlighted. Worldwide, an estimated 9 to 30 million unplanned pregnancies occur annually as a consequence of contraceptive failure. The frequency of failure of contraceptive methods highlights the continuing need for abortion services." (WHO speaker at a Royal College of Obstetricians and Gynaecologists held April 1995, reported in G. Penney, 'Induced Abortion: the next decade', *Brit. Journ. Obs. & Gyns.*, 1995: 103;754-756)

[7] These included Dr Helena Wright, Stella Browne, Janet Chance, Alice Jenkins, Dr Norman Haire, Dora Russell, Nurse E.S. Daniels and Lord Horder, 1st President of the National Birth Control Association.

[8] See Chapter Three.

[9] "...from the moral point of view contraception and abortion are *specifically different evils*: the former contradicts the full truth of the sexual act as the proper expression of conjugal love, while the latter destroys the life of a human being; the former is opposed to the virtue of chastity in marriage, the latter is opposed to the virtue of justice and directly violates the divine commandment "You shall not kill". (*Evangelium Vitae*, 1995)

Chapter One:

FROM MALTHUS TO MARIE STOPES.

The birth controllers, their motives and methods; the opponents of birth control; the apparent success of birth control; the falling birth rate; the sexist nature of birth control; how history has been re-written.

The prevention of conception is dramatically different to abortion. Opinions on the importance of each one as a social and ethical issue tend to differ. The two lobbies are, naturally enough, seen as distinct from each other, and vague notions of historical origins suggest two separate campaigns.

And yet, the pamphlet *Abortion: The struggle in the Labour Movement* contradicts this assumption: "Although the struggle for a Woman's Right to Choose appears to have developed recently it has in fact grown naturally out of the broader struggle for women's rights, in particular the right of women's access to contraception as a means of fertility control."[1]

From this, the student of birth control history naturally concludes that the fight for abortion sprang from the struggle for women's rights, with the early feminists and socialists. In fact, the abortion rights movement did not begin until well into the twentieth century, after full adult suffrage had been granted, and long after the first feminists and socialists had unfurled their banners (and, in some cases, furled them again). But the latter part of the statement is true. The abortion campaign *did* spring from the campaign for birth control.

To trace the real beginnings of the birth control movement, we must go back a little further in history - not quite to the dawn of time, as birth control historians would suggest - but to the closing years of the eighteenth century.

Birth Controllers: their Motives and Methods

One of the earliest and best-known advocates of birth control was Anglican parson Thomas Robert Malthus. His *Principle of Population*, published in 1798, insisted that population increases in geometric ratio (2,4,8,16), whereas the food supply increases in arithmetic ratio (2,3,4,5). Put simply, he believed that population would always be ahead of food provision. Prior to Malthus and his theory, and — more importantly - the first National Census of 1801, there were no reliable figures for population, and there was a widespread belief that it was actually declining. In those days, a thriving population was associated with national wealth and well being. (A not-dissimilar belief exists in many poorer countries today).

However, Malthus disagreed. He believed that unless population growth was restricted, man was doomed to poverty. It is probable that millions of poor people have lived and died without ever hearing the name of Malthus. But he was to have a profound and lasting effect upon their lives, and upon our own.

For a century, Malthus' theory was used by economists and policy-makers to justify *laissez-faire* (non-interventionist) economic policies; it even underpinned the English Government's lukewarm response to the Irish famine.[2] According to historian G. Talbot Griffiths, opponents of social or economic reform argued that it was useless for governments to try to help the poor. No matter what society did to relieve poverty, they said, numbers would inevitably increase, outstripping provision. Any help given would only encourage the very poverty it was trying to relieve. In the same philanthropic vein, destruction of empty cottages was seen as a good way of discouraging early marriage, and promoting emigration.[3]

Malthus blamed the Poor Law for promoting population growth, as he thought it encouraged the poor to have more children by its payment of children's allowances.[4] In his *Second Essay*, he went so far as to question the poor man's right to existence:

"A man who is born into a world already possessed, and if he cannot get subsistence from his parents on whom he has a just demand, and if the society do not want his labour, has no claim of right to the smallest portion of food, and, in fact, has no business to be where he is."

This philosophy laid the foundation stone of the population control campaign. From now on, some would hold the poor responsible for their own poverty, simply by being alive; consequently, the only answer to the problem of poverty was that the poor should not be born.

Malthus advocated late marriage, abstinence and workhouses, where "fare should be hard", in order to curb the numbers of the poor, as well as public works and private luxury investment. He saw this as the only alternative to the traditional curbs on population - war, famine and pestilence. Instead of being killed outright, the poor would be prevented from coming into existence by preventing their parents from coming together.

Was Malthus right? Talbot Griffiths points to the reduction in mortality as a cause of rising population.[5] In other words, people were living longer, so there were more alive to count. However, as he points out, Malthus was so convinced of his theory that he never adequately set out his premises, or examined their logical status. Nor did he handle factual and statistical materials with much critical or statistical rigour, despite the great developments being made in this field during his time. Though he was adamant that, without control, population would swamp the earth, he had no idea of the amount of unused land available.[6]

As Bernard Schreiber points out, forecasting population increase was difficult, without any population increase or food production statistics to rely upon. On what then, did Malthus base his ideas? Solely, according to Schreiber "...on some small travels and minor observations".[7] Nevertheless, his mathematics, geometrical explanations and diagrams had a "hypnotic effect". Few questioned his theories. Most significantly Malthus, living up to his nick-name ("Gloomy"), never took into account the fact that human ingenuity, begetting new technology, could overcome seemingly intractable problems of subsistence. Perhaps he was unfamiliar with the old adage that necessity is the mother of invention.

Peter Fryer, in *The Birth Controllers*, alleges that Malthus 'borrowed' his theory of population from other sources.[8] Despite this, as commentator Garret Hardin demands: "Why can't we forget Malthus, though every year he is 'proven wrong and buried - only to spring to life again before the year is out'. If he is so wrong, why can't we forget him?"[9] Perhaps the answer is that we want him to be right. As Schreiber points out, Malthus sought a biological remedy for an economic problem. It is far easier to blame the victim of an economic system, than to change the system.

This may provide a clue to Malthus' anxiety. The eighteenth century was a century of revolution. The 'natural order' was being overthrown in France and the Americas, with Tom Paine proclaiming 'The Rights of Man'.[10] The spectre that haunted Malthus was not famine and pestilence, but democracy. What would happen when all those who had "no claim of right to the smallest portion of food" began to press that claim through the ballot box?

His *Essay on the Principle of Population*, written anonymously in 1798, was Malthus' attempt to refute the utopian doctrines of philosopher William Godwin. For Godwin predicted unlimited progress for mankind, with the sweeping away of old reactionary institutions. Malthus attacked Godwin for not caring "...how many children a woman had or to who they belonged."[11] Godwin's response was for man to embrace "moral restraint" as an answer to the 'population problem'.[12]

Samuel Johnson, with more insight into poverty than the formidable Parson, remarked: "It is not from reason and prudence that men marry, but from inclination. A man is poor; he thinks, 'I cannot be worse, and so I'll e'en take Peggy.'"[13] Percy Shelley saw a great social threat in "sophisms like those of Mr Malthus, calculated to lull the oppressors of mankind into a security of everlasting triumph". Karl Marx was a little more blunt, condemning Malthus' "reactionary tendencies", and calling him "contemptible" and a "shameless sycophant of the ruling classes".[14]

The family allowances paid under the Speenhamland System of outdoor relief, and blamed by Malthus for encouraging large families, were abolished by the 1834 Poor Law. The new Law established the workhouses. These places, dreaded by the poor, were to be forever associated with Dickens' *Oliver Twist*. They fulfilled a secondary function by segregating the sexes, thus preventing poor people from begetting more children. The poor now had to fend for themselves, and the slow battle for workers' rights began, giving rise to the organised labour of the Trade Union movement.[15]

As a champion of the poor, all Malthus could offer was fewer poor people. His views sprang, not from a dream of women's liberation, but from a nightmare vision of democracy. But although Malthus himself did not advocate contraception - a fact that historians frequently mention as an interesting quirk of character - later disciples of his Theory did.

Malthus may have had a horror of contraception, but those who followed him had no such scruple. However, there was no organised body of thought or opinion on the subject of population and birth control until late in the nineteenth century, only a handful of individuals inspired by Malthus. Who were these individuals, and were they any more sympathetic to women than the gloomy parson had been?

The early birth control advocates were all male. Their ideas were not popular; indeed, they were exceedingly *un*popular in some quarters. They were certainly not part of a popular campaign.

According to Peter Fryer, what little birth control agitation there had been, died down during the 1840s. There was acute unrest in the country following widespread industrialisation, and its accompanying evils; the poor trudged from the countryside to the mushrooming industrial cities, and made their homes in jerry built slums. Voting was still in the hands of a privileged few, and 'rotten boroughs' (where a tiny electorate returned a representative to Parliament, while thousands living in sprawling industrial towns had no representation), were common. In Dorset, a small group of poor agricultural labourers took a secret oath, formed a trade union, and were transported for treason. The treatment of the 'Tolpuddle Martyrs', as they became known, caused uproar.

The Chartists took up the banner of social reform and they, like William Cobbett, opposed Malthusianism.[16] Neither did Malthus' ideas – if they heard of them - seize the imagination of the poor, concerned only to survive. There were riots and street battles, and some of the hated workhouses – fruits of Malthus' dream - were pulled down.

There was a great deal of birth control propaganda, but it was mostly thinly disguised advertisements for condoms. And yet, many birth control advocates were radicals, like Francis Place (1771-1854), a self-educated man who had suffered poverty. He helped draw up the People's Charter after which the Chartists were named, and fought against the persecution of the trade unions. He supported birth control in the belief that it would help the poor by reducing their numbers, thus giving them greater bargaining power. He himself had a large family (15 children, of whom five died in infancy), and he felt the irony of his own example of 'moral restraint'. His views on contraception made him unpopular, however, and many of his acquaintance shunned him for this reason. Later accounts of his life barely mention this aspect of the great radical.

Richard Carlile (1790-1843), a friend of Place, was also of humble origins. He initially found birth control abhorrent, but was converted by Place. Carlile published radical books, such as Tom Paine's *Rights of Man* and *The Age of Reason*. In 1817, there was a clampdown on the radical press. Carlile was frequently arrested and imprisoned for defending insurgent agricultural labourers, but was still convinced that the main evils of the day were bad government and the priesthood. He wrote *Every Woman's Book; or What is Love?* claiming, "bastard children, deserted children, half-starved and diseased children, badly-housed families - all were a tax upon love". Better to use preventives than abortion and infanticide. He, like Place, recommended that women use the contraceptive sponge, despite the "initial shock to the female mind".

This exhortation to women, from a man impatient with their annoying sensibilities, was to find many an echo as the birth control movement got into its stride. However, it does illustrate the shocked response of most women to birth control, with its implications for their status as women. After all, the only women who used such methods were prostitutes and, it was said, rich women who wished to cheat on their husbands.[17]

The early condoms were not designed to prevent inconvenience to women, but inconvenience to men. Commonly known as 'preventives', they were worn to protect men against acquiring sexually transmitted diseases (STDs) from prostitutes, who supplied them to customers, as did brothels. It is likely that the contraceptive 'side-effect' was welcome to prostitutes because pregnancy was a hindrance to their trade. It was also inconvenient for brothel-keepers because it represented lack of income.

Another birth control advocate was John Stewart (1749-1822), a kind of early health-freak, who warned against damp sheets and recommended coarse soap as a preventive against STDs. In old age he practised *'coitus reservatus'* (sex without climax), not because of any consideration for women, (it is hard to see how this method could be of any benefit to women, since it involved a prolonged act of intercourse until, presumably, the man fell asleep), but to conserve his 'vitality' while still indulging himself.

Robert Dale Owen (1801-1877), son of pioneer industrialist Robert Owen, wrote *Moral Physiology: or A Brief and Plain Treatise on the Population Question*, which was devoted to the social and eugenic arguments for family limitation. Owen immigrated to America where he caused consternation among emancipators by voting against prohibition of slavery in newly acquired American territories.

American physician Charles Knowlton (1800-1850) wrote the notorious *Fruits of Philosophy*, which was to prove instrumental in establishing the birth control movement in Britain. He argued that conception control would prevent overpopulation, hereditary disease, and preserve and improve the species. He also claimed that it would reduce the numbers of artificial abortions and infanticide.

Women's Issues?

Birth control in the nineteenth century *was* associated with women's emancipation - but the idea came, not from women, but from men. Eminent British philosopher John Stuart Mill (1806-1873), wrote *On the Subjection of Women* in 1869. But in *Principles of Economics*, published in 1848, he had *already* linked the question of women's liberation with birth control. He assumed that the 'evil of overpopulation' would diminish as women achieved greater freedom. He was not the first political thinker who realised that to check the birth rate women must be ideologically harnessed to the view that political freedom meant freedom from children. However, their delicate sensibilities would have to be roughened up, like the knees of unfortunate climbing boys, in order to check the population.[18]

In fact, William Thompson (1775-1833), pioneer of British socialism and the co-operative movement argued in his *Appeal of One Half of the Human Race*[19] that political rights were the prerequisite of domestic and civil rights. He anticipated that in a "free and equal society", "women might be expected to show greater prudential foresight and thus with the emancipation of women the problem of population pressure would disappear."[20] Interestingly, the rejection of woman as 'breeding machine',[21] associated with feminist criticism, was originally a male idea. It is unlikely that women of the time – including feminists - looked upon themselves in that light.

Thompson, however, had a low opinion of domestic virtues, which spilled over in references to women's "slave-like mentality", and their being "confined, like other domestic animals" to the house, with a "…tendency to attach too great …importance to domestic and selfish over social and sympathetic affections…" Thompson held that children, though important, should "never be allowed to interfere with more socially useful functions". What about pregnancy? He supplies the answer: "…should women freely participate in political activities for men" at an age when they were "liable to such casualties as childbirth", birth control should be made available to them.[22]

Perhaps it was dawning on such activists, that without biological 'liberation', there would be no one to make the tea at political meetings. However, at the time, such ideas were not popular with men or women, a fact noted by birth control historians Joseph and Olive Banks.[23] They observe that in the 1830s and 1840s, many new women writers appeared who emphasised not contraception, but women's domestic duties.

The Neo-Malthusians

The ideas of Malthus won little popular support in a nation where many poor people struggled to survive, straining to hold on to the barest essentials of life. One false move would send them plunging into an abyss of financial ruin and misery vividly portrayed by social commentator and artist Hogarth and his Victorian successors.

Society was composed of many strata. Below the upper class (the landed and titled gentry) was the many-layered middle class: professional men, doctors, lawyers and clergy. There were also wealthy tradesmen. Below them were shopkeepers, teachers and clerks; below these, the working classes: shop workers; skilled men and tradesmen. Further down, the manual labourers, the unskilled, the casual labourers. Below these, the completely indigent, surviving no one knew how. There were great numbers of homeless children, babies abandoned at birth and armies of domestic servants.

This mass of population would probably have had Malthus spinning in his grave. But after the 1870s, something strange happened: the birth rate began to fall. This coincided with a famous obscenity case, the Bradlaugh and Besant trial of 1877. Charles Bradlaugh was a well-known political figure, a radical who was elected to Parliament as a Liberal in 1880, but for six years refused to take the oath of allegiance to enable him to take his seat. Annie Besant was the estranged wife of a clergyman. She led the famous 'Match girls strike' at Bryant and May in 1888, fighting for better conditions. With Bradlaugh, she published Charles Knowlton's *Fruits of Philosophy,* mentioned earlier. The book was considered obscene, and a prosecution ensued. The resultant publicity has been widely credited with alerting the public to the advantages of birth control.

Both Bradlaugh and Besant were disciples of Malthus. Bradlaugh formed the Neo-Malthusian League, and propounded Malthus' gospel in his periodical, the 'National Reformer'.[24] However, when Mrs Besant converted to theosophy, she renounced her views on birth control. She spent the latter part of her life in India, where she worked for Indian independence. After Bradlaugh's death in 1891, interest in Malthusianism waned.[25]

It was left to Dr George Drysdale, who had written articles on Malthusianism for the *National Reformer,* and published an anonymous book on birth control, to pass on the torch to his brother Charles Robert Drysdale, who was to become President of the League. For the next forty years, the League would be a Drysdale dynasty, with Charles Robert being succeeded by his wife, Alice Vickery Drysdale, and later his son, Dr Charles Vickery Drysdale, ably assisted by *his* wife, Bessie Drysdale.

The League was financed by the Drysdales until its 'demise' in 1927. Over the years, Drysdale money paid for the printing and distribution of over three million publications.[26] But despite the falling birth rate, the Malthusians were not popular. One Annual General Meeting attracted only five members and supporters.[27] It was the Drysdale money that kept the campaign alive.

The chief reason for this unpopularity was their propaganda. It was repellent, and succeeded in antagonising practically everyone. It was to be expected that their frank advocacy of birth control would attract criticism, and for many years they claimed that they did not publish instructions on practical birth control because they feared to offend.

This fear, however, did not extend to offending people politically, and in every other way. Their economic views echoed those of conservative economist Adam Smith and, as historian Richard Soloway says, though claiming political neutrality, they were "rabidly anti-socialist".[28] They held that overpopulation was responsible for wars and poverty. A fall in the birth rate, they claimed, would lead to a fall in the death rate and prosperity and peace. They also claimed that the fear of begetting children forced men to resort to prostitutes. When challenged with the possibility that men could (and should) remain celibate, they detailed an alarming list of the injurious side effects of celibacy.

Birth control, they claimed, would enable men to marry early - thus avoiding prostitutes and sexually transmitted disease - complete their small family, and prosper. Their assumption that men could not be chaste offended many people - not least feminists, who argued that it was men, not women, who needed to change their ways.

Realising that their cause needed to be popularised, Charles Vickery Drysdale copied the outdoor meetings of socialists, and was encouraged by the results. But when the Great War started, the Neo-Malthusian League fell from grace, and their arguments suffered a credibility loss from which they never really recovered. They advocated a moratorium on births, arguing that, since wars were caused by overpopulation, a cessation of births was the only way to peace. This enraged opinion in a country that lost millions of men in combat.[29]

After the Second World War, Margaret Sanger, the American birth control advocate, arrived in England. She too called for a moratorium on births. She too met with an angry response.[30] It was clear that Sanger, who had earlier referred to "battalions of unwanted babies",[31] regarded such babies as the real enemy. Their arrival in the world must be prevented at all costs, and gave sufficient reason not to mince her words.

Malthusian ideas, which on closer examination proved to be nonsense, like bad smells, have lingered. After the recent Rwandan conflict, in which thousands were butchered, a letter printed in the *Independent* newspaper called for birth control for the refugees.[32] This theme was taken up in the run-up to the Cairo Conference on population, by Edward Luce and John Hooper: "Total wars, which target civilians of all ages, leave behind more evenly distributed populations. Rwanda and Cambodia both fall into this category. If the Cambodian example is anything to judge by, then Rwandans – including the Tutsis – will stage a rapid reproductive recovery over the next few years."[33]

More recently, the Marie Stopes International group caused a storm by sending contraceptives to Kosovan refugee camps, although most women were separated from their men due to the conflict. It may seem incredible that people who have lost loved-ones in war should be faced with demands not to have children, but it does at least give a clue to the Malthusian philosophy. This philosophy understands very little about the reasons for having children, seeing every normal human act as the result of either rational thought, rather like a commercial transaction, or instinct, like animals. It is as confused about bereavement, and human attachments, as it is about the motivations for bringing new life into the world. It has little sympathy for individual human beings, because it sees human beings as the problem.

Demands for moratoria on births sprang, not from compassion, but from cold calculations. In the great mysterious sea of human population, it is well known that there is a surge of births following a war. This is what the Malthusians feared. They argued that it was sheer madness to squander the gains made in war (i.e. the reduction in the population) by producing more human beings after the war was over. Evidently this philosophy lives on.

Though latter-day disciples of Malthus had some strange ideas about population, their arguments were well criticised at the time, and their wildest claims exposed as nonsense. As early as 1825, Cobbet, who railed against

Malthus, in his *Rural Rides*, pointed out that the earth would always provide "sustenance and sufficiency" to all those given their "fair share of its products".[34]

How then, did the Neo-Malthusians sustain their belief that 'population' was a problem? Did they believe their own rhetoric – or was there another purpose to their campaign? Their spiritual leader, Parson Malthus, did not believe in contraception, classing it with other "methods of vice" such as abortion, infanticide and *coitus interruptus*. He saw it as a "sexual perversion",[35] and recommended instead late marriage and abstinence. As we have seen, however, the Neo-Malthusians had a horror of celibacy.

The abhorrence Malthus felt for contraception is often referred to in a joking aside. How ironic, that a movement dedicated to the spread of artificial birth control, should have as its patron saint a man who deplored artificial birth control! For *Neo*-Malthusians (as they called themselves), however, contraception was essential, for they had discovered sex as an enjoyable pastime. George Drysdale, writer of *The Elements of Social Science*, regarded sex as both pleasurable and health giving.[36] However, unrestricted sex would lead inevitably to children, which would frustrate the aims of population control.

This fear of begetting children who would be dependent on the paternal purse would also, it was said, interfere with male pleasure. A woman's pregnancy meant the frustration of her husband's sex drive for several months at least. Prostitutes, though expert in avoiding pregnancy, also gave disease. The use of a 'preventive', it was also claimed, interfered with male pleasure. The only answer was to instruct respectable women in female methods of contraception.

The tiny band of Neo-Malthusians hi-jacked Malthus' name, therefore, in order to propagate contraception as the pre-requisite of (male-centred) recreational sex. They were convinced that once men became 'converted' to this view, they would also be converted to contraception (this is why indecent pictures were used in conjunction with birth control literature), thus enhancing human happiness (male, at least) without an increase in the population. But there were many obstacles standing between them and those annoying, respectable women.

The Opponents

It was to be expected that the Church would be opposed to the preaching of the birth control gospel. After all, was not marriage instituted "for the begetting of children"? Christian society saw contraception as a horrifying abuse of a wife's sensibilities by her husband, encouraging him to treat her like a common prostitute. Virtue in women was seen as laudable, and Christian men were expected to try to live up to this ideal, too. Jesus Christ was, after all, the ideal role model for celibate men.

The approval of birth control also seemed to fly in the face of trust in God to provide for the children he sent. Unease was not officially voiced - perhaps because of embarrassment as to the subject matter - until well into the twentieth century. In 1914, however, placing Victorian delicacy firmly behind them, a committee of Bishops issued the 'Misuse of Marriage' document, which condemned contraception, commended the 'safe period', but excused from fault those women whose husbands insisted on using contraceptives.[37]

The 1920 Lambeth Conference condemned 'unnatural means', and warned of the dangers of contraception, and of sex being seen as an end in itself.[38] When a birth control clinic, the Birmingham Women's Welfare Centre opened in 1927, a protest petition launched by the Archdeacon of Birmingham was signed by 54 clergymen.[39] The Bishop of London's campaign to stop the sale of contraceptives by chemists was aided by the all-denominational United Public Morality Council.[40]

It was the opposition of Catholics, however, which the birth control advocates found most worrying. Their arguments were not substantially different from the other Christian denominations, but they had firmer leadership. In 1930, a papal encyclical condemning (among other things) contraceptives, *Casti Connubii,* was issued.[41] More importantly, Catholics held positions in the medical services and in local government, which made them obstacles in the way of any birth control plan. They also played a large part in the Labour Party – more of which later.

Medical opposition to birth control was a serious problem for the Malthusians.[42] Doctors were vocal in their criticism. Their authoritative warnings of the dangers of contraception[43] were seriously upsetting to those who would spread the gospel of birth control.

Warnings of sterility and mental instability may resemble quaint Victorian warnings against masturbation, but that is how many people of the time regarded contraception. They believed that it enabled couples to, in effect, masturbate each other, rather than joining in a loving relationship, sharing responsibility for any resulting children.[44] They also believed it was a man's duty to abstain from sexual demands on his wife if she was too ill to have children.

Such strokes of fate were commonly regarded as giving people the opportunity to achieve virtue through suffering, rather than using suffering as an excuse to behave badly.

There was no lack of opponents – especially medical - for the birth controller to reckon with, and - contrary to what may be supposed - they were not all male and Catholic. The League of National Life was an interdenominational organisation formed in 1926, to combat the spread of contraceptives. By 1929 it had 560 members.[45] Medical opponents included the pioneering woman doctor, Elizabeth Blackwell.[46]

It should be borne in mind, too, that there was another aspect to contraception that caused much concern. Female methods were very similar to methods of abortion, for example, syringing after intercourse; the 'sponge', (recommended by Besant and Place); the 'Dutch cap' (pioneered by the Malthusian Dr Aletta Jacobs in Holland). All these introduced foreign objects into the woman's body. There was quinine, too, recommended by some birth controllers as a douche, or later, a suppository, which could also be used as an abortifacient.[47]

Such connotations were strenuously denied by the Malthusians, who began to stress that their object in spreading contraceptive 'knowledge' was precisely in order to avoid the 'need' for abortion. Their rejection of such fears as ignorant, however, was on a par with their dismissal of *any* opposition to their beliefs. This attitude was glaringly evident throughout the pages of their periodical, the *Malthusian.*

From the beginning, socialists had objected to Malthusianism.[48] As Fryer points out, Francis Place realised as far back as 1824, that it was important to gain the ear of the working classes, because of their "hatred for Malthus the mountebank-parson (as Cobbett dubbed him)." The poor "were convinced that the purpose of Malthus' 'Essay' was to exalt the rich and debase the poor...his arguments were used by landowners as an excuse for clearing their estates of peasants."[49]

At the beginning of the nineteenth century, radical agitators speaking on behalf of the poor knew from their own experience how the rich used the arguments of Malthus to exploit them. By the end of the century, labour was organising itself into Trade Unions. The poor had at last gained a voice of its own. There was a growing realisation among birth control advocates that if Malthusian propaganda was to succeed, it had better address the needs of the poor, and from 1880, *The Malthusian* was sub-titled "A Crusade Against Poverty". But its virulent anti Labour stance angered socialists.

The Malthusian argument that large families were the cause of poverty, clashed head-on with the socialist view that poverty was the fault of the economic system, not the poor. Unfortunately for the Malthusians, the politicised poor were fairly good at recognising anything that reeked of Malthus. An ounce of their experience of hardship was, to them, worth far more than a ton of Malthusian theorising. Family limitation was seen, at best, as a personal matter, and at worst, as an attack on a poor man's right to children.[50]

Labour Party members were 'emotionally repelled' by the idea of contraception,[51] and perhaps this was not surprising, given the attitude of middle-class Malthusians to working-class sexuality. In their eagerness to represent their campaign as a compassionate one to 'end poverty', the Malthusians portrayed the poor as little better than beasts who could not control themselves and, in the absence of contraception, would go on begetting children whether they could afford them or not.[52]

A new sensitivity towards feminism (which was becoming more vocal), softened this lurid picture somewhat, and they began to lament the fate of 'poor women' at the mercy of unintelligent, loutish men - a picture still fresh today, but one which hardly endeared itself to the working men the Malthusians wished to convert. In reality, however, the Malthusians hoped, not to free women from the demands of men, nor to free the poor from the demands of children, but to free society from the demands of the poor.

Neo-Malthusians with socialist contacts tried to convert them to birth control, but with little success. However, Annie Besant (more successful than most), found compassionate arguments for birth control were more favourably received by her left-wing friends.[53] The Social and Democratic Federation, for example, was 'antipathetic' to the idea - probably because, as Audrey Leathard notes, birth control activists were "totally middle class".[54] But if socialists were antagonistic to birth control, surely feminists were in favour?

Monstrous Regiment of Women

Richard Soloway argues that the early feminists concentrated their campaigns on single women and widows. Few questioned the maternal role. Birth control was not an objective of the organised women's movement until well into the twentieth century. Even after the First World War, feminists continued to spurn the subject.[55]

Joseph and Olive Banks point out that the organised women's movement concerned itself with specific abuses, e.g. the franchise, sex barriers in education, etc.[56] Their reasons for non-involvement in – even hostility to - the birth control movement - would startle and dismay some modern feminists. Although they did not consider large families essential, they equated a woman's right to control her own body, not with the right to use contraceptives, but with the right to refuse sex.[57]

In an age that suffered from a shortage of eligible men, the idea of celibacy gained popularity with Victorian and Edwardian feminists - an alarming development, no doubt, to the Malthusians who apparently regarded access to women's bodies as a right safeguarded by the use of contraception. In response to an enquiry, C. V. Drysdale remarked: "Many spinsters would, no doubt, see great merit in polygamy".[58]

Far from seeing polygamy as the answer to their problems, however, the feminist movements in Britain and the United States saw contraception as another form of male oppression and rejected it. They feared it would encourage another form of 'polygamy' - extra-marital sex - thereby corrupting marriage and undermining women's solidarity.[59] With remarkable prescience, they foresaw a situation in which a transformation of women's sexual *mores* would not guarantee freedom for women, but would make it possible for some women to 'poach' other women's husbands.

The early feminists have been excused by modern commentators for their apparent reluctance to become involved in the birth control campaign (of the leading feminist publications, not one mentioned the 'famous' Bradlaugh and Besant trial),[60] with suggestions that they feared to endanger the fight for the franchise, or simply that they were too prudish to discuss sex.

Joseph and Olive Banks dismiss the suggestion that the Victorian feminists were reluctant to associate themselves with campaigns relating to sex. They point to the energetic support for Josephine Butler's campaign against the compulsory examination of prostitutes for Venereal Disease; also for the campaign to raise the age of consent for girls, in order to stamp out sexual abuse. They suggest that the feminists' problem was not that they could not *discuss* sex, but that they were *anti*-sex.[61]

The most cursory examination of Victorian feminism reveals that Victorian feminists were not shrinking violets. Their fight for justice for women was inspired, in part, by the abuse of female sexuality by a minority of men. They saw contraception as just another form of sexual abuse. They argued that, once the fear of creating dependent children was removed by contraception, more women would be open to more abuse. The element of male self-control and responsibility necessary in a married relationship would decrease. Contraception would liberate men, not women.

With a continuing drop in the birth rate, ironically it was feminists who were accused of a 'flight from motherhood'. They defended themselves by asserting that it was not the politically active woman who despised motherhood, but that the move towards small families was motivated by the selfishness[62] of the 'socially emancipated' woman, who contributed nothing whatever to feminism.[63] A particularly outspoken feminist, Frances Power Cobbe, who had exposed the extent of wife beating and torture in England, railed against 'emancipated' women's licentiousness, lack of chastity and adultery.[64]

The 'Woman Question' was indeed central to the movement to control births because - quite simply - it is women who produce babies. If the birth control movement was to succeed, it was *women's* fertility that had to be controlled at all costs. In this respect, a certain imbalance in the sexes was not to be deplored, since it meant fewer women to reproduce. This - not a respect for women's autonomy - was the root of Drysdale's opposition to polygamy.[65]

Despite evidence such as this, Claire Tomalin, biographer of feminist Mary Wollstonecraft, states: "There remains the question as to why more women did not welcome the early birth-control campaigns, and the answer to this looks like deliberate, persistent and villainous suppression by the established male preserve of Church and State." However, for further information, she suggests "Peter Fryer, *The Birth Controllers*... and N. Himes, *Medical History of Contraception*..."[66] Neither represented a female viewpoint; Himes was part of the birth control movement, as we shall see.

At Last - A Popular Movement?

Newspapers and magazines tended to reflect the public's distaste by not giving birth control a high public profile - despite the insensitive efforts of Malthusians. Delicacy of feeling towards the young, difficult to appreciate now, dictated caution in the discussion of matters which implied that children were unwelcome burdens, responsible for poverty and misery. But in 1877, the obscenity trial against Bradlaugh and Besant at last ensured wide publicity for the Malthusian cause. And in 1880, a little-marked event took place that ensured birth control would become, if not famous, at least infamous: Marie Carmichael Stopes was born.

Stopes, and her American counterpart Margaret Sanger, have been credited with 'popularising' birth control. Stopes was a doctor, not of medicine, but of philosophy, a brilliant palaeontologist, whose 1918 book *Married Love* was a huge best seller. She opened her first birth control clinic in the Holloway Road in London in 1921. By 1935, 66 local authorities were giving birth control advice, and 47 voluntary clinics had been established.[67]

By the 1920s, birth control was being debated in the political parties and the women's organisations. According to Marie Stopes, women were flocking to her clinics in their thousands. Several birth control advocacy groups had sprung up, including Stopes' own birth control organisation, the Society for Constructive Birth Control and Racial Progress. There was even a Workers' Birth Control Group.

Opposition from feminism and medicine seems to have faltered, and in 1930, the Church of England's Lambeth Conference, which ten years previously had warned of the dangers of artificial contraceptives, condemned contraception only for selfish reasons.[68] The culmination of the process was not reached until 1958, when family planning was finally endorsed by the Conference,[69] but from a casual glance at history, it would seem that birth control had finally 'arrived'.

From being a tiny, isolated and deeply unpopular group with sordid connotations, birth controllers were at last seen to be holding centre-stage, their opponents reduced to carping from the wings. It all seems too good to be true. Perhaps this is because it was not true. Birth control had not really become respectable enough to be discussed over most peoples' tea tables, or even over the garden fence[70]. But there *was* debate in political organisations - those organisations that had formerly ignored, or outright rejected birth control. How had this happened?

How had opposition from socialists, feminists, medicine and the church - all serious obstacles to the aims of population controllers - been removed? The answer to this puzzle is that the obstacles were not removed, but the opposition of the organisations in question was weakened from within by members whose first allegiance was to birth control. To use modern feminist parlance, the birth controllers were 'specific issue antagonists,'[71] who devoted their time and energy to achieving prominence for the birth control issue, using the machinery of their chosen organisations to do so.

Birth control clinics were formed; but as we will see, the numbers of women visiting them were tiny, even allowing for possible embarrassment, ignorance, or fear. Seeing the success of public health campaigns for sanitation and clean water, birth control advocates realised they could only reach the poor (and have the kudos of a public health campaign), by insisting that birth control advice be made available at local authority Mother and Baby clinics. (This 'advice' would be, in the first instance, simply to direct poor women to the nearest voluntary clinic. Eventually they hoped that the clinics would actually give the birth control advice, at public expense.) Consequently, agitation within the Labour Party was aimed at forcing the Ministry of Health to allow local authority clinics to give such advice.

After a monumental battle within the Labour Party, the Ministry of Health quietly issued an official memo in 1930, permitting birth control advice to be given for health reasons. It seemed that the battle had been won. By 1939, all the birth control advocacy groups - with the exception of Stopes' organisation – had joined together, and become known as the Family Planning Association.[72]

The Fall in the Birth Rate

As we have seen, the birth rate began falling during the 1870s. It took a few years for this phenomenon to become clear. When it did, many different theories were produced to explain something that had never happened before, something that many in society found deeply worrying, because a thriving population had traditionally been associated with national strength and prosperity.[73]

The Neo-Malthusians did not hesitate to claim credit (which probably did nothing to enhance their popularity, since a fall in the birth-rate was not seen as a good thing), pointing to the publicity engendered by the Bradlaugh and Besant trial.[74] It was obvious, they proclaimed, that newspaper accounts had aroused interest in, and desire for, contraceptive knowledge. Some agreed - those both for *and* against contraception. Their claims have been echoed by modern birth control historians.[75] But were they right? There were many other factors at play, which may account for the drop in the birth rate, and which did not necessarily include the sudden and widespread use of methods previously deemed repellant.

The nineteenth century was a time of vast improvements in public health. The industrial revolution, with its verminous and insanitary jerry-built housing, open sewers and infected water supplies - not to mention the terrible working conditions of men, women and children – had had a disastrous effect on the health of the poor. Children were born in the slums, and died in them, in great numbers. Any poor woman, should she be lucky enough to see her family to maturity, would expect to lose some on the way. Poor nutrition meant lack of resistance to common illnesses. Doctors cost money, and were called in only as a last resort. In the slums, 'preventive medicine' was letting children play in the dirt to build up their immunity.[76]

Artificial infant feeding, resorted to by poor women forced to work outside the home, brought with it the dangers of over-dilution, contamination, and poor nutrition, and played a part in the horrific toll of infant mortality.[77] A reduction in breast-feeding also dealt a blow to a natural method of conception control which helped 'space' children.[78] More babies were born, and more died.

Even the wealthiest of couples marrying in the 1850s and 1860s lost between 20 - 30 per cent of their children.[79] As for the poor, E. P. Thompson states that of every thousand children aged up to five years born in industrial towns, over half died.[80]

However, between the years 1905 and 1938, the Infant Mortality Rate dropped from 130 per thousand to 55.[81] As more children survived, the birth rate began to drop, from a mid-Victorian average of six children per family, to 3.4 in Edward's reign, to under three by the outbreak of the First World War.[82] Queen Victoria, who herself had nine children, raised all of them to maturity. But well-to-do families of nine or ten were becoming less and less common.

Improvements in public health meant that the infant mortality rate began a steady decline. The terrible epidemics that started in the slums and claimed their victims even in the upper classes (Prince Albert died of typhoid in 1861) began to ease their terrifying grip on the imaginations of the comfortably off. A child born in the slums, however, might still be easily 'carried off' by a contagious disease like scarlet fever, diphtheria, or even the measles.

The dangers to poor children from working were lessened, as industrial legislation progressively curtailed the employment of children in factories. This meant that they could no longer be used as cheap, expendable labour. The Education Act of 1870 ensured elementary education for all children, up to age twelve. These factors might lead to the conclusion that children had, by the late nineteenth century, become more of an economic liability than an asset, possibly giving parents a financial incentive to practise fertility control.

However, child labour in the home came free, and when poor mothers needed an extra pair of hands to help with a new baby, older daughters were often called upon. Additional children did not represent lack of earnings to women, since most married women did not work if they could help it. And for the poorer classes, there were no school fees to consider, and no legacies to divide between the offspring. When they grew old enough to leave school at twelve years old, they could contribute to the family purse. Children were still an economic asset to the poor.

Poor people looked to their children to care for them when they got old - the horror of the workhouse to the indigent poor loomed large, well into the twentieth century.[83] But in 1908, the first old age pension was introduced by a Liberal government. Though tiny, it gave the elderly poor a modicum of independence. As people looked forward to a more secure old age, and a longer life span, the need to rely on many children grew less urgent, and families got progressively smaller.

The poor, then, had no educational costs, no patrimony to divide, and depended on their children's support in old age. They were less likely to see children as financial burdens. Wealthier parents, on the other hand, saw private education as an investment, ensuring their children a professional career and a good income in adulthood. This, they hoped, would provide their children with the means to uphold their standard of living. School fees were expensive, however, so middle-class parents might have been inclined to limit their families to one or two children instead of five or six.

Olive and Joseph Banks, themselves birth control advocates, reject the myth that birth control was historically a feminist objective, and conclude that, in an age when men held the purse strings, it was men who dictated the size of the family. They suggest that birth control was utilised for economic reasons.[84]

However, this being the case, the poor would have had even more incentive than the rich to limit their families. But in all areas - infant mortality, age expectancy, disease and physical development - there was a marked difference between the classes. This became a matter of concern for those interested in public health, politics, or social affairs. Soloway writes: "Pointed questions about the physical quality of the race had been raised at the time of the Boer War both within parliament and without...disproportionately large numbers of recruits from industrial towns... were unable to meet minimal physical requirements for military service..."[85] This led in 1904 to a government enquiry into 'Physical Deterioration'.[86]

But for the Malthusians, the greatest problem was not the deaths of so many poor children, but the birth and the survival of so many poor children. They had identified a problem that filled them with alarm. It was the differential birth rate.

While the neo-Malthusians boasted of their success in lowering the birth rate by the spread of contraceptive information,[87] it was becoming apparent that their perceived success did not extend to the slums. It was not necessary to consult statistics and graphs, to see that poor families were large, and well-to-do families small. The 'campaign against poverty' was more successful, apparently, with those who were *not* poor. If, as has been alleged, it was the better-off sections of society that utilised birth control because of their greater knowledge of such methods, it is interesting that those most concerned with the falling birth rate - the members of the self-appointed National Birth-Rate Commission - were able to boast on average only 1.75 children each.[88]

Radiant Motherhood

The ever-widening gap between the classes, expressed in health, longevity and physical development, and now in family size, brought with it a strange social cleavage. As middle-class families grew smaller, the nature of the family and parenting changed. While motherhood was still exalted, fewer and fewer women were becoming mothers - and those who did, were mothering fewer children. Advice to mothers proliferated, and new classes of professional 'mothers' came into being.

As Ann Oakley remarks in *Housewife*: "Until late in Western history the only experts in childcare and child behaviour outside the family were the midwife and the teacher. Now the world is full of experts."[89] A dizzying array of professions was expanded by the childcare industry. Teachers, psychologists, doctors, nurses, social workers, inspectors, writers, social pundits - and birth controllers - all knew how to bring up children. Though such 'mothers' may not have had to qualify for such status by actually giving birth, the surrogates did not hesitate to bestow their knowledge on a generation of women grown too nervous, by a dwindling experience of young children, to trust their own instinct.

Childcare, from being the prerogative, and the unchallenged territory, of individual mothers for centuries, became a battleground for different theorists. As the birth rate decreased, children became the focus of everyone's attention - except when it came to practicalities. At the end of the day, it was still mother who was left holding the baby, even though she might not be sure what to do with it.

Psychiatrist Sigmund Freud stressed the relevance of childhood to adult mental conditions. His theories have been called into question,[90] but the new emphasis on childhood - not just as something to be physically survived, but to be managed so as to ensure *mental* survival - became widespread. Unfortunately, some new childrearing methods were as damaging to children as the old repressive Victorian ways.

In his book 'The Mechanical Baby',[91] Daniel Beekman describes the inhuman regimes devised by childcare 'experts' (often men), in the quest for the perfect baby. Bowel-training, feeding, washing, all were to be done to a rigid' timetable, with as little contact between mother and child as possible. Crying was to be ignored; thumb-sucking and masturbation, rocking and head-banging (often the only comforts left to an infant with little human contact), were to be severely dealt with, using such ingenious instruments of torture as cardboard, leather or aluminium cuffs; tapes, and bitter-tasting substances on the fingers and thumbs.

Dr Luther Emmett Holt, in *The Care and Feeding of Children*, writing in 1894 about the harm done by playing with very young babies, warns: "They are made nervous and irritable, sleep badly and suffer from indigestion..." Holt, a popular author on childcare, states baldly: "Never give a child what it cries for."[92]

Were these strict regimes devised for the baby's welfare? Or were they devised for the comfort of the adults? It is more likely that babies, nature's supreme anarchists, had to be tamed in order to promote the smooth running of the household. Domestic chaos was inimical to the rigidly ordered middle-class man, who probably suffered from an inability to control his own working life. Home was to be a haven from the world of business, and with the new emphasis on companionate marriage, children, with their arbitrary and apparently illogical demands were bound to get in the way.

Instead of babies being regarded in the traditional way as gifts from God, they were to be treated as objects of production, with the mother as the manager, directed by a surrogate mother - the professional baby expert.

Babies, designed in a sophisticated way to ensure their survival by making their demands clear in the only way they know how, were to be treated like the blank pages of a book. Unless they were taught how to behave by adults, apparently the world would be peopled by nappy wearing, thumb sucking, foot stamping, men and women. Instead of mothers being taught the needs of the child *by the child*, they were taught (against their own instincts), to teach the child how to behave. Middle-class mothers, anxious to rear their babies in the best possible way, were eager for professional advice.

Even women who bravely rejected such advice where it seemed to conflict with their child's well being, found their confidence in their own mothering instinct undermined. This particular form of 'mother's help' succeeded in demoting mothers from the most important, to the least important, person in the child's upbringing.

Breast-feeding, so important in building up babies' resistance to disease and allergy - and the last thing a mother could do that the professionals could not – came to be seen as inferior. The practice of bottle-feeding grew among middle-class mothers, assured by the professionals that they 'did not have enough milk'. Breast-feeding was seen as second best, something to be resorted to by those who could not afford powdered milk. Diarrhoea, constipation, colic and other problems, arose to plague the harassed mother, making motherhood burdensome.

Even playing with a baby was done in obedience to instructions to stimulate mental development. Though borne willingly, having children was not a burden to be borne too often. The birth rate continued to decline, and with it, the status of mothers. Smaller families did not produce healthier babies; neither did they automatically turn women into better or happier mothers.

What has been portrayed as a movement to help mothers (and, by tortuous reasoning, children), ended in benefiting neither. It was built on the rationale that fewer is better, a rationale not employed in any other area of human activity (especially not in the area that obsessed the Neo-Malthusians: sex). This should not really be surprising, given the attitude of many birth controllers. From the very beginning, little attention was paid to women's welfare.

Writing in 1745 to a young friend "on the Choice of a Mistress", Benjamin Franklin gives eight reasons for preferring old women to young ones. Beginning with complimentary remarks on their "conversation", Franklin goes on to more important matters: "...there is no hazard of children, which irregularly produced may be attended with much inconvenience."

He also advises that older women are "more prudent and discreet in conducting an intrigue" and would prevent a young man "ruining his health and fortune among mercenary prostitutes." Franklin goes on: "The face first grows lank and wrinkled; then the neck; then the breast and arms; the lower parts continuing to the last as plump as ever: so that covering all above with a basket, and regarding only what is below the girdle, it is impossible of two women to tell an old one from a young one. And as in the dark all cats are gray, the pleasure of corporal enjoyment with an old woman is at least equal, and frequently superior; every knack being, by practice, capable of improvement."

It is not to be thought that Franklin had no thought for women's welfare in all this, however. He finishes: "8th and lastly. They are so grateful!"[93] Franklin was exercised by the population 'problem', writing in 1755: "Was the face of the earth...empty of other inhabitants, it might, in a few ages, be replenished from one nation only, as, for instance, with Englishmen."[94]

Casanova, like Franklin, was complimentary in his 'commerce' with women, exclaiming gratefully: "There is no need for harlots in this fortunate age. So many decent women are as obliging as one could wish."[95]

It is not to be supposed that all such men, detailing their experience of 'condoms, cundums, or condums' (references to which, according to Peter Fryer, in his survey of 17th Century English literature onwards, were made by the male customers of prostitutes and brothels), were lacking in compassion towards women. In the 1720s, White Kennett, son of the Bishop of Peterborough, wrote a poem extolling the liberating effects of the condom on young women, thus freed from the fear of "big Belly, and the squawling Brat".[96]

Not all men favoured the condom, however. According to Dr George Drysdale, brother of the first President of the Malthusian League, the condom "dulls the enjoyment, and frequently produces impotence in the man and disgust in both parties..."[97] He goes on: "Any preventive means, to be satisfactory, must be used by the woman, as it spoils the passion and the impulsiveness of the venereal act if the man have to think of them."[98]

It seemed that, for a small minority of men to enjoy sex, women were required to be not only constantly available for sex, but also used as a repository for anything whatsoever introduced into their bodies for the purpose of avoiding the "hazard of children, irregularly produced". Casanova, when not using condoms made of fish membrane, recommended half a lemon inserted in the vagina.[99] Francis Place recommended the 'sponge' to women, despite the "initial shock to the female mind",[100] so that sex might be made "independent of the dread of conception".[101]

Whether this dread was men's, or women's, is not clear. Place certainly dreaded the consequences of overpopulation, blaming poverty on it. Now, it seemed, the age-old excuse for women rejecting a sexual relationship (fear of pregnancy), was to be done away with. F0rom now on, there would be no excuses.

Modern Methods

As we have seen, some methods of contraception were confused with abortion - and for good reasons. The campaigning journalist W. T. Stead, in 1899, admitted practising, "...simple syringing with water. Of late always withdrawal."[102] However, other ingredients could be used, for example, vinegar,[103] recommended by Charles Knowlton in *Fruits of Philosophy*.

Later, Marie Stopes would recommend quinine douches.[104] In their pamphlet *Hygienic Methods of Family Limitation*, published in 1913, the Malthusian League recommended, amongst other delights, douching with vinegar, citric acid, permanganate of potash, or hydrogen peroxide. Showing a touching solicitude for women's comfort, they add that this could be done without the wife leaving her bed, if there was a second tube to carry away the liquid, or a bedpan.[105]

But if syringing was to be carried out efficiently, it implied the co-operation – at the very least - of a partner. In describing Knowlton's syringe, modern author Fryer shows unconsciously how what has been reconstructed as a 'feminist' act of fertility control, actually carried overtones of sexual violence. Knowlton recommended a syringe with a soft metal barrel and a piston head made tight with a wrapping of tow, to be used within five minutes of emission. Orders were clear, with no thought spared for female sensitivities: "The woman should assume the right position and introduce the syringe deeply into the vagina."[106] Thus the completion of the sexual act was not a cuddle, a kiss, or even a cigarette, but a cold, heavy, metal object.

The indifference of early birth controllers to the discomfort, pain, disgust and fear, which must have been felt by women using these 'methods' is matched by that of modern commentators on the subject. There is no lack of evidence, but rather a reluctance of commentators to acknowledge that this was a campaign fought by men, for men.

Though some writers, to their credit, have noted the ghoulish preoccupation with women's physiology in the quest for the perfect contraceptive,[107] most seem to regard the cruel eccentricities of the birth controllers as a cause for amusement. This implies a disturbing inability to accept that women were actually experiencing, not liberation, but exploitation.

Norman Himes (who refers to the Marquis de Sade as an "eighteenth century writer")[108] relates how Casanova took a dozen condoms to try out on a fifteen-year-old servant girl, to ensure their quality, before embarking on an affair with a "public woman".[109] Perhaps allowances should be made for 1930s writers such as Himes; however, even in the 1960s, Peter Fryer relates amusing anecdotes of the women of ancient Egypt inserting crocodile dung into the vagina as a contraceptive,[110] and the ancient Japanese using hard sheaths made of tortoiseshell horn or leather.[111]

Referring to the practice of douching, Fryer remarks: "Done immediately after coitus, it was fairly reliable but rather troublesome."[112] He even quotes de Sade who, in his *La Philosophie dans le boudoir*, lists his favourite methods of birth control, including the vaginal sponge, the condom, but most of all, anal intercourse as "la plus delicieuse, sans doubte", but reassures us that we need not take the third method "too seriously".[113]

William Brennan, in *Studies in Prolife Feminism*, describes the writings of de Sade as consisting of "...a heavy diet of sex, torture, and killing inextricably intertwined". In the pornographic novel *Justine*, "the victimizer takes time out from his brutal assaults against his female victims to express serious doubt whether 'this peculiar creature, as distinct from man as is man from the ape, had any reasonable legitimate pretensions to classification as a human."[114] There were other methods of 'fertility control', of which de Sade also approved. These were abortion and infanticide, which will be examined later.

Such practices are repeated for the reader's edification, while the social dynamics that must have been involved (violence, coercion, economic dependency and exploitation), are not touched upon.[115] It seems probable that these ancient 'methods' were used by prostitutes who, unlike other women, were not expected to bear children.

Malthus, for example, considered that prostitution - along with poverty, war, disease and a high death rate - were necessary to keep down the population.[116] The Neo-Malthusians were convinced that there would be no need of prostitutes if only wives would use contraception. In this, there was a veiled threat to women that if they did not use contraception their husbands would resort to the brothel.[117] Prostitutes, after all, existed for the convenience of others, and as such, were not accorded the human right of physical integrity.

It is clear from the attitudes of birth controllers, and their bizarre array of birth control appliances, that women were being used as guinea pigs in the quest for population control, the various methods having been first tried on prostitutes.[118] The Neo-Malthusians certainly felt confident enough to publicise their economic theories to the respectable public in countless handbills, and to advertise manufacturers of birth control appliances in their periodical. But since the respectable public would not read their propaganda, they had to look for other means.

How History was Re-written

The Bradlaugh and Besant trial has been seen (variously) as a fight for the right to knowledge,[119] by two courageous birth control protagonists;[120] a triumph for free speech,[121] and for the right to publish helpful information without running the risk of being prosecuted for obscenity.[122] The motives for prosecution have been given as the rich selfishly keeping contraceptive knowledge to themselves;[123] the fear of sex;[124] the right-wing fear of the poor obtaining contraceptive knowledge. (!)[125]

In a summing-up typical of the commentary available, Joseph and Olive Banks hint that, though sales of the controversial book rocketed as a result of the trial, and 'everyone' wanted birth control information, the subject was still 'taboo'.[126] The episode is presented as though there was a fund of secret knowledge available only to the rich and powerful. The birth controllers only needed to 'unlock' the treasure trove, and so make it available to the poor.

Were Bradlaugh and Besant simply a couple of hapless philanthropists, persecuted by the authorities on behalf of a prudish establishment, whose motive was fear of the working classes discovering sex? On the contrary, from first to last, the publication of Knowlton's *Fruits of Philosophy* was a calculated attempt by the pair to establish the right to publicise birth control free from the fear of prosecution.

In 1876, *Fruits of Philosophy* had been the subject of an obscenity prosecution in Bristol.[127] Henry Cook, a bookseller, received two years' hard labour,[128] the pages of the book having been interleaved with indecent plates. In January 1877, the London publisher was charged with publishing an indecent book, pleaded guilty, and the book was seized by the police.[129] Bradlaugh and Besant decided to publish the book themselves, although it had circulated freely among Malthusians for 40 years.

Their intention was to provoke a test case, which would ensure that birth control literature could be disseminated among the public without legal hindrance.[130] The pair took a shop behind Fleet Street in London, in order to republish the book, with medical notes by Neo-Malthusian Dr George Drysdale.[131]

The newly printed copies of the book were stored at Bradlaugh's home, while he paid a visit to Scotland. Fearing a police raid, Mrs Besant and Bradlaugh's daughters hid copies "in every conceivable place" – some were even buried in the garden.[132] On his return, Bradlaugh, not wishing to appear ridiculous, insisted they be retrieved.

A copy was despatched to the chief clerk of the Magistrates at the Guildhall, with a formal notification that the book would be on sale in Stonecutter Street the following day, from four to five. A polite request was sent to the Detective Department, that they be arrested at some hour convenient to both parties. A third notice was delivered to the city Solicitor, whom they expected to lead the prosecution.[133] To their disappointment, the would-be birth control martyrs were not arrested immediately, but were forced to cool their heels until April, when they were remanded on bail.

The case was transferred to the High Court, and in a five-day trial, Dr C. R. Drysdale, (brother of George, and later to be President of the Malthusian League), gave evidence on their behalf.[134] Bradlaugh and Besant were accused of obscene libel, i.e. of disseminating matter calculated to destroy or corrupt the morals of the people. Bradlaugh and Besant defended themselves by arguing that the book was not obscene, and the birth control practices it advocated were in the best interests of humanity.

It is recalled by birth control historians as an afterthought, that Besant had such a low opinion of the forty years out-of-date *Fruits of Philosophy*, that she shortly after published her own treatise on birth control, entitled *Laws of Population*.[135] Far from helping humanity, their aim was to help the birth control movement spread its message.[136] Ironically, while the jury found the defendants guilty under the law for publishing the book, they exonerated them from corrupt motives.[137] The truth was, the book which the two Neo-Malthusians had gone to such trouble to publish, was worthless - and dangerous - rubbish.

Massachusetts's physician Charles Knowlton wrote his contentious book in 1832. As a young man, he received two months' imprisonment for stealing a corpse from a graveyard and dissecting it.[138]

Considering that he obtained his knowledge of physiology in such sensational ways, his knowledge of the human female reproductive system was negligible. He thought the human egg took four weeks to travel down the tube to the uterus. He described the uterus, ovary and tube, as one-third too small, with the cervix projecting into the vagina one-third too far. He greatly overestimated the secretion of vaginal mucous, and saw menstruation as a preparation for conception, rather than evidence that conception had not occurred. He thought the average age of menopause was 45, rather than 49.[139]

Knowlton was the first physician to describe the vaginal douche.[140] He recommended solutions of alum, and other astringents - hemlock, red rose leaves, green tea, raspberry leaves or roots, zinc and baking soda - apparently for their spermicidal qualities.[141] Sugar of lead, he suggested, could be useful for (not surprisingly) any "tenderness".[142]

Writer Elizabeth Draper comments: "Other nineteenth-century American writers advocated tannin, opium, prussic acid, iodine, strychnine, alcohol and carbolic...Some of these were obviously dangerous and many of them if used in too strong solution could irritate or damage the delicate membrane of the organs, thereby sometimes preventing conception from this unwanted cause. Little was known about the quantities needed and some writers failed altogether to instruct how their recommendations should be carried out."[143] It is obvious that methods intended to be contraceptive might end up sterilising any woman unfortunate enough to experience them.

Knowlton suggested that the vagina should be syringed two or three times after male emission, with a liquid that would dislodge nearly all the semen, and destroy the potential of any that remained.[144] His inclusion of cold water as a spermicide,[145] and the recommendation that "...five minutes' delay would not prove mischievous - perhaps not ten,"[146] demonstrate his lack of knowledge.

Clearly indifferent to any physical damage (quite apart from mental and emotional distress) caused by his favourite method, Knowlton boldly proclaimed: "Any publication, great or small, mentioning the syringe (or anything else that operates on the same principle) as a means of preventing conception - whatever liquid may be recommended, is a violation of copyright".[147]

Like Knowlton and others, Annie Besant's recipes for douches were alarming, and obviously the product of guesswork. Frequently they were far too strong for safe use, and instructions sometimes suggested that the 'patient' should reduce the quantities if irritation occurred.[148] Besant, in *Laws of Population*, gives a detailed prescription for the use of alum or sulphate of zinc, made into a solution to be used in the syringe, also a sponge soaked in a solution of twenty grains of quinine to a pint of water. Himes, writing in 1930s, says that quinine (*besides* being irritating to some women) was of low spermicidal power.[149]

Though the birth controllers treated opposition and criticism with contempt, they themselves were far from being experts. Even the celebrated Annie Besant knew the unreliability of the methods she recommended. In *Laws of Population*, she warns: "there is much uncertainty attending the use of all these injections."[150] She was constantly revising her work in its several editions (though with information just as unreliable), and pleaded for more medical knowledge on this "intricate subject".[151] This sounds remarkably familiar even today, as old methods are discredited, and every new method hailed as a 'breakthrough'.

Despite this, according to Soloway, the writings of Charles Knowlton and George Drysdale "formed the scientific core of the Malthusian League's propaganda...".[152] Interestingly (in view of the fact that neither Bradlaugh nor Besant were medically or scientifically qualified), in 1880, the second objective of the newly-formed Medical Branch of the League was: "To obtain a body of scientific opinion on points of sexual physiology and pathology involved in the 'Population Question', and which can only be discussed by those possessed of scientific knowledge'.[153]

Nevertheless Norman Himes, writing in the 1930s, says of the Bradlaugh/Besant trial: "Millions of people learned of more effective methods."[154] Sales of the book - like any publication deemed to be obscene - were indeed high,[155] but it is doubtful whether it would be of any use to those wishing to learn "effective methods". Besant herself admitted, in Laws of Population: "If the spermatazoa have entered the womb before the injection is used, conception may occur..."[156] If anything, the methods advocated would be more likely lead to an upsurge of unplanned pregnancies.

However, as Himes remarks: "There can be no doubt that the publicity gave wide advertising to the idea that contraception was possible".[157] Clearly, the motivating force behind these two birth control advocates was not compassion, but population control.

It is curious that Bradlaugh and Besant, with their professed concern to alleviate the suffering of the human race by curbing births, could deliberately promulgate outdated and misleading information, which would be more likely to lead to unplanned pregnancies. If the birth controllers were missionaries, intent on winning converts, it would appear that their own private religion was more important than the welfare of those they were trying to help.

Probably they reasoned that, even if these methods were not always effective, they might at least work some of the time, so were of some use. This view would agree with the population controllers' preoccupation with numbers. Any birth averted was, to them, a success, regardless of any discomfort, pain, or distress caused to their 'flock'.

With even the 'experts' on mechanical contraception so ignorant, what about other, more natural methods of birth control? Germaine Greer, in Sex and Destiny, argues that these methods were already employed but, strangely, the Malthusians warned against them.

It was known that there was a 'safe period' during the female cycle when infertile intercourse could take place.[158] There was 'coitus interruptus', where withdrawal took place before the male climax. There was the strange practice of '*coitus reservatus*' already mentioned. There was good old-fashioned celibacy. In addition, nursing a child could act as a natural 'spacing' of children.

All these were, in turn, either condemned by the birth controllers, or damned with faint praise.[159] Besant, for example, refers to the 'safe period' as "not certain", but withdrawal as "absolutely certain as a preventive".[160] However, she recommended a small wad of cotton to be used by females as a preventive, to be worn during the day and removed at night. She also condemned prolonged nursing of infants, quoting at length a popular medical writer, Dr. Chavasse, on the injuries allegedly inflicted by this practice.

There was much ignorance and confusion over what constituted the 'safe period' (of which more later). Once again, through their ignorance, the birth controllers risked actually *boosting* the numbers of unplanned pregnancies by giving worthless advice.

We return full circle to the puzzle of why those apparently anxious to limit births should condemn these methods, and especially the most reliable method of all - abstinence - while simultaneously promulgating the most unreliable methods. To discover the answer, we must go back to the Godfather of the Malthusian League, Dr George Drysdale, and his insistence on the use of female birth control methods only.

Writing in 1854, he denied that contraception would lead to moral evil, saying abstinence was far more unnatural, and "totally incompatible with health and happiness". The book was called, appropriately, 'Physical, Sexual and Natural Religion', but later editions were entitled 'Elements of Social Science'. It was published anonymously, and dedicated to "the poor and the suffering", a "trumpet blast" against abstinence, prostitution and poverty. On his deathbed, Drysdale implored his brother, Charles Robert, to press unceasingly for State regulation of the size of families.[161]

Significantly, what the alternative methods of birth control, such as the 'safe period', or abstinence, had in common, was that men would have to abstain from the sexual act or (as with *coitus interruptus*), give up some part of the pleasure to ensure that conception did not take place. Sex had become of primary importance to George Drysdale and his followers. To them, it *was* a religion.

Traditionally, self-control exercised in the cause of a loved-one's comfort was seen as noble. Any husband who insisted on 'conjugal rights' at the expense of a sick wife's health would have been condemned. Sweethearts who were parted could show the depth of their devotion by their steadfastness and fidelity in separation, and husbands and wives could show the depth of *their* devotion by steadfastness and fidelity in marriage. A man who did not break off his engagement when his fiancee became sick or injured was admired as a hero.[162]

The Malthusians' notion of man's sexual gratification at all times, stemming from their belief that sexual fulfillment was necessary for his physical and mental health, was completely foreign and abhorrent to the culture at which they preached. And, despite Soloway's claim that the Neo-Malthusians, like all good Victorians, believed in hearth and home,[163] George Drysdale, in *Elements of Social Science*, gives a flat contradiction of the rosy picture, stating: "Marriage distracts our attention from the real sexual duties, and this is one of its worst effects."[164]

What were these mysterious "real sexual duties"? According to Drysdale: "Marriage is based upon the idea that constant and unvarying love is the only one which is pure and honourable, and which should be recognised as morally good. But there could not be a greater error than this. Love is, like all other human passions and appetites, subject to change, deriving a great part of its force and continuance from variety in its objects; and to attempt to fix it to an invariable channel is to try to alter the laws of its nature."[165]

His views would certainly have been at home in the 1990s; in the 1890s, he was not so fortunate. In 1899, Dr Elizabeth Blackwell, the first woman to qualify in medicine, remarked: "Here, in this chief teacher of the Neo-Malthusians, the cloven foot is fully revealed. This popular author, who in many parts of his book denounces marriage as the enslavement of men and women, who sneers at continence, and rages at Christianity as a vanishing superstition, all under a special pretence of benevolence and desire for the advancement of the human race, here clearly shows what he is aiming at, and what his doctrines lead to. Male sexual pleasure must not be interfered with, male lust may be indulged in to any extent that pleasure demands, but woman must take the entire responsibility that male indulgence be not disturbed by any inconvenient claims from paternity. Whatever consequences ensue the woman is to blame, and must bear the whole responsibility." She concludes:

"A doctrine more diabolical in its theory and more destructive in its practical consequences has never been invented. This is the doctrine of Neo-Malthusianism."[166]

George Drysdale's brother Charles claimed that the "small family system" would not only end poverty and the social misery of overpopulation, but would eliminate "sexual diseases" such as prostitution and celibacy. This would be accomplished by young men marrying early, thus avoiding the clutches of diseased prostitutes and the misery of sexual abstinence. Apparently, they would have children early, and then avoid having more by the use of contraception.

This optimistic view was not shared by Richard Carlile, who feared that the greatest preservation of chastity in women was the fear of pregnancy, and if this could be avoided by the use of contraception, it would lead to the "breaking up of all individual attachments". According to Carlile, who was converted to contraception after an initial abhorrence, love was a disease whose only cure was requitement - distressing and disastrous only if not cured. Discarding romantic pretences altogether (and apparently oblivious to one half of the human race), he bluntly declaimed: "The passion of love is nothing but the passion to secrete semen in a natural way".[167]

The Neo-Malthusians ridiculed medical warnings against contraception,[168] while doctors saw the problems caused by its after effects. The Senior physician to the Samaritan Hospital for Women and Children, Charles Henry Felix Routh, warned that wives practising contraception faced the prospect of contracting (variously) metritis, leucorrhoea, menorrhagia, haematocele, hysteraligia, and hyperaesthesia of the genital organs to galloping cancer, ovarian dropsy, ovaritis, sterility, nymphomania and the possibility of suicide. Men might face nervous prostration, mental decay, and loss of memory, intense cardiac palpitations and also a tendency to suicide.[169] Some symptoms appear far-fetched. However, if the douches recommended by the Malthusians were followed, they must have caused severe damage.

As time went on, the doctors admitted their ignorance, but were still reluctant to recommend contraception in case of possible harm.[170] The Neo-Malthusians, however, never admitted *their* ignorance, and in their turn, listed some strange side effects they claimed were associated with alternative methods of birth control. George Drysdale, for example, condemned *coitus interruptus* as "...physically injurious, and... apt to produce nervous disorder and sexual enfeeblement and congestion, from the sudden interruption it gives to the venereal act, whose pleasure moreover it interferes with."[171]

The Neo-Malthusians (unlike Malthus) regarded celibacy as a 'curse', resulting in "peevishness, restlessness, vague longings and mental instability in men and chlorosis and hysteria in women".[172] Charles Robert Drysdale, in 1879, castigated the Church for condemning poor parishioners to unnatural celibacy or impractical, joyless abstinence – presumably for not preaching about contraception.[173]

George Drysdale, for his part, denied that contraception would lead to moral evil, saying abstinence was far more unnatural, "totally incompatible with health and happiness, producing the "most widespread and desolating diseases". In fact, he saw 'preventive intercourse' as "the only possible way of introducing real morality into human society".[174] In case anyone should think that the terrible physical side-effects of celibacy might be worth risking, in order to win *spiritual* brownie points, Drysdale warns: "Chastity, or complete sexual abstinence, so far from being a virtue, is invariably a great natural sin".[175]

By constantly harping on the duty of sexual enjoyment, the Neo-Malthusians must have exacerbated, rather than helped those whose only option was to remain celibate. Their writings, rather than improving sexual relationships, encouraged the idea of looking for someone to satisfy sexual tastes developed in isolation.

One correspondent of the *New Generation*, bemoaning his bachelor state (he had, since boyhood "practised continence or self-denial in sexual matters"), claimed celibacy had caused him "almost indescribable harm in both body and mind...played havoc with my whole nature and constitution, and...reduced me to a nervous wreck." While admitting the evils of "promiscuous intercourse", he pleads: "...what about the other evil of going without the experience altogether...?"[176]

The Safe Period

While natural alternatives to contraception were invariably condemned by the population controllers, their knowledge of these methods - as well as the methods they actually recommended - was highly unreliable. The 'safe period' is an example of something improperly understood, which was nevertheless recommended. George Drysdale, for instance, thought the 'safe period' was 2-3 days before a period, to eight days after it.[177] Besant also refers to the 'mid-period'.[178]

Another Malthusian, Dr Allbutt, thought the 'safe period' to be five days before, and eight days after, menstruation.[179] In 1913, the Malthusian League issued a pamphlet entitled 'Hygienic Methods of Family Limitation', giving the 'Safest Period' as the "middle fortnight between the monthly periods".[180]

Not until the First World War was it realised that the majority of soldiers' wives who became pregnant did so within twenty-one days of their menstrual period. As Soloway remarks: "The findings seemed to disprove the long-held assumption that the 'safe period' came in the middle of the monthly cycle and that maximum fecundity peaked just before menstruation in harmony with female passion. It had always seemed logical that, in accordance with natural selection, the 'period of desire in women should be the likeliest time for conception', and as this occurred at the beginning of the cycle the risk of pregnancy should have been greatest at that time".[181]

Dr Dinnie Dunlop and Stopes were eugenicists, hence the interest in 'natural selection' and the 'mating' of the human species. Dunlop's stunned realisation (he apparently "professed expertise on the subject"),[182] that what had been hitherto recommended as safe was actually *unsafe*, did not affect the birth controllers' dispensation of 'knowledge'. They continued to consider themselves experts.

NOTES

[1] Pamphlet, Labour Abortion Rights Campaign. (Undated, circa 1978)

[2] In his essay Population, Malthus argued: "The land in Ireland is infinitely more peopled than in England; and to give full effect to the natural resources of the country, a great part of the population should be swept away from the soil." (In David Alton, *Life after death: Britain's tragic abortion story 1967 – 1997*, The Christian Democrat Press, 1997, p75)

[3] G. Talbot Griffiths, *Population Problems, of the Age of Malthus*, Frank Cass & Co Ltd, London, 1967. (First published 1926, Cambridge University Press)

[4] J. P. Huzel, quoted in Edwin Brooks, *This Crowded Kingdom*, Charles Knight & Co., 1973, p36.

[5] Population Problems of the Age of Malthus, *op cit*

[6] See Bernard Schreiber, The Men Behind Hitler: A German warning to the world, tr. H. R. Martindale.

[7] *ibid*

[8] Sir James Steuart, Robert Wallace, Josiah Townsend, and others; in *The Birth Controllers*, Secker & Warburg, London, 1965

[9] *Population, Evolution and Birth Control: A Collage of Controversial Ideas*, ed. Garrett Hardin, W. H. Freeman & Co., San Francisco, 1969, 2nd ed., p3.

[10] Published 1791.

[11] *Population, Evolution and Birth Control, op cit*, p16.

[12] *ibid*, p188. Godwin did not, however, follow his own prescription for moral restraint, believing in the liberty of the individual in most matters.

[13] *ibid*, p33.

[14] *ibid*, p69.

[15] See E. P. Thompson, *The Making of the English Working Class*, Penguin, England, 1984.

[16] See Peter Fryer, *The Birth Controllers*, Secker & Warburg, London, 1965.

[17] In her biography of Mary Wollstonecraft (*op cit*), Claire Tomalin suggests that the "greater sexual enthusiasm of French women and prostitutes probably rested on their command of a simple birth-control device: the sponge." (p.138) Tomalin, who relies heavily on Fryer's work, claims: "The sponge was not wholly reliable, but had the great advantage of simplicity – French women were reputed to wear one attached to a ribbon tied round the waist – and of course control by the woman herself." If this rumour were true, it would probably not have encouraged respectable English women to follow suit; if it were *not* true, its circulation might merely demonstrate the low opinion of English women for such practices. Once again, the efficacy of the method takes second place to 'female control' which, if economic realities and power relations are left out of the discussion, is probably meaningless, and 'sexual enthusiasm', real or imaginary, the true goal.

[18] See Olive Banks, *Faces of Feminism*, Martin Robertson, Oxford, 1981; *Abortion: The struggle in the Labour Movement* (*op cit*); See Richard Soloway, *Birth Control and the Population Question in England 1877-1930*, Chapel Hill University North Carolina Press, 1982; Joseph & Olive Banks, *Feminism and Family Planning in Victorian England*, Liverpool University Press, 1964.

[19] Published in 1825 – see *Feminism and Family Planning in Victorian England, op cit*.

[20] W. Thompson, *Practical Directions for the Speedy and Economical Establishment of Communities, on the Principles of Mutual Co-operation, United Possessions and Equality of Exertions and of the Means of Enjoyment*, Cork, 1830.

[21] Thompson, *Appeal of One Half of the Human Race, op cit*.

[22] *Ibid*

[23] See *Feminism and Family Planning in Victorian England, op cit*.

[24] *Feminism and Family Planning in Victorian England, op cit*, p6.

[25] For many years, the Malthusian League had no office, a tiny income, and membership of barely one hundred. (*The Birth Controllers*, p74).

[26] See *Birth Control and the Population Question in England 1877-1930, op cit*.

[27] *The Birth Controllers, op cit*, p74.

[28] *Birth Control and the Population Question in England 1877-1930*, op cit.

[29] Within days of the outbreak of hostilities, [Charles Vickery] Drysdale alarmed by frantic cries for more children to compensate for anticipated losses, proclaimed the young a burden on the nation's limited resources. With the nation facing untold demands and its men a perilous future, it was foolish, he argued, to encourage women, many of whom will soon have no reliable means of support, to assume the obligation of raising children alone." *Malthusian*, August 1914, p64;

September 1914, p71; December 1914, pp89-90; in *Birth Control and the Population Question in England 1877-1930*, p74.

[30] She arrived in June 1947. (See Audrey Leathard, *The Fight for Family Planning*, Macmillan, 1980, p82)

[31] M. Sanger, *Family Limitation* (31st edition)

[32] "Rwanda is the most densely populated country in Africa, with an alarmingly high rate of population growth.... The only feasible economic solution is an effective programme of family planning in Rwanda." (Letter, dated 17 May 1994, from Oliver Knowles (former adviser to the Communaute Economique des Grands Lacs) These, and similar views, were later refuted by Rakiya Omaar, of African Rights, in a letter to the *Guardian.*

[33] In demographers' terms, the Rwanda slaughter is a mere blip: overpopulation is what worries the experts. EDWARD LUCE and JOHN HOOPER examine their hard logic as the United Nations prepares for its Cairo conference next month." (*Guardian,* 13.8.94)

[34] William Cobbett, *Rural Rides*, Everyman edition, pp52-53, in *Life after Death op cit.*

[35] *This Crowded Kingdom*, Charles Knight & Co., 1973, op cit, p24.

[36] *The Birth Controllers, op cit,* p2.

[37] *The Birth Controllers, op cit,* p240.

[38] *ibid,* p243

[39] *The Fight for Family Planning, op cit,* p38.

[40] *The Birth Controllers, op cit,* p243.

[41] 31st December 1930. It excluded the 'safe period' from prohibition.

[42] See *Birth Control and the Population Question in England 1877-1930, op cit,* Chapter Six, *Medicine and Malthusianism.*

[43] Dr Halliday Sutherland, *Birth Control*, Harding & More Ltd., London.

[44] French doctor L.F.E. Bergeret's *Conjugal Onanism* (1868) was frequently cited (see Jeffrey Weeks, *Sex, Politics and Society: the regulation of sexuality since 1800*, Longman, 1989, p45)

[45] See *Birth Control and the Population Question in England 1877-1930*, and *The Birth Controllers.* The League's president was Dr Frederick J. McCann, a prominent gynaecologist; vice-presidents were Charles Gore, a retired Anglican Bishop, Joseph Hertz, the Chief Rabbi, and Dr Mary Scharlieb. The League was begun by Dr Halliday Sutherland and Dr Laetitia Fairfield, both Catholic converts; Lord Hugh Cecil and Edward Lyttelton were also supporters.

[46] Birth Control, *op cit,* p99.

[47] See Barbara Brookes, *Abortion in England 1900-1967*, Croom Helm, London, 1988.

[48] See *The Fight for Family Planning*, p29; though by the 1930s, the correspondence and advertisement columns of the left-wing *Daily Herald* seemed to buck this trend. (*Control of Life,* p95)

[49] *Essays on the Principle of Population addressed to the Working Classes*, in The *Birth Controllers*, pp72-73.

[50] *Faces of Feminism, op cit,* pp187-8.

[51] *The Fight for Family Planning, op cit,* p29.

[52] See *Birth Control and the Population Question in England 1877-1930, op cit.*

[53] *Birth Control and the Population Question in England 1877-1930, op cit,* p84.

[54] *The Fight for Family Planning, op cit,* p29.

[55] *Birth Control and the Population Question in England 1877-1930*, op cit.

[56] *Feminism and Family Planning in Victorian England, op cit,* p26.

[57] Faces of Feminism, *op cit*, p76.

[58] *New Generation*, November 1923, p135.

[59] *Faces of Feminism, op cit*, p74.

[60] *Birth Control and the Population Question in England 1877-1930, op cit*, p134.

[61] See *Feminism and Family Planning in Victorian England, op cit*.

[62] *Feminism and Family Planning in Victorian England, op cit*, p121.

[63] *ibid* p105.

[64] *The Contemporary Review*, 1878, in *Studies in Prolife Feminism*, Vol.1, No.3, Summer 1995.

[65] "...but we are satisfied that the actual development will be in other directions." (*New Generation*, November 1923, p135)

[66] Tomalin, *op cit*, p.308.

[67] See The Fight for Family Planning, *op cit*.

[68] *The Birth Controllers, op cit*, pp245-6.

[69] *ibid* p268.

[70] See *The Birth Controllers,* pp185, 179 and 311n; Peter Fryer discusses how birth control knowledge is thought to have spread, in the absence of any firm evidence.

[71] This term is usually reserved for pro-life feminists; see Robin Rowland, *Women Who Do and Women Who Don't Join the Women's Movement*, Routledge Kegan Paul, London, 1984.

[72] See *The Fight for Family Planning, op cit*.

[73] See *Birth Control and the Population Question in England 1877-1930,* for discussion on the various theories; factors as diverse as the rising age of women on marriage, women's education, better nutrition, urban life, and the advance of civilisation, were blamed. Thomas Doubleday's anti-Malthusian theory, resurrected by James Barclay, rested on cyclical-nutritional theories – in short, the better the nutrition, the smaller the birth rate.

[74] Dr Halliday Sutherland, *Control of Life, op cit*, p92; *Birth Control, op cit*, p75.

[75] See The Birth Controllers, *op cit*, Chapter 17; Feminism and Family Planning in Victorian England, *op cit*, pp91-2.

[76] A doctor's advice to my maternal Grandmother in respect of my Uncle Leonard, now in his eighties.

[77] See Elizabeth Roberts, *A Woman's Place: An Oral History of Working-Class Women 1890-1940*, Basil Blackwell, Oxford, 1985.

[78] See Germaine Greer, *Sex & Destiny,* Pan Books Ltd., London, 1985.

[79] Fertility of Marriage Census, in *Birth Control and the Population Question in England 1877-1930,* p44.

[80] *The Making of the English Working Class, op cit*, p361.

[81] Infant Mortality Rate and its Components, in Jane Lewis, *The Politics of Motherhood*, Croom Helm, 1980, p32; see also *Abortion in England 1900-1967, op cit*, p49 n.129.

[82] N.L. Tranter, Population since the Industrial Revolution: The Case of England & Wales, New York, 1973, p98, in Birth Control and the Population Question in England 1877-1930, p7.

[83] In the 1920s, my Mother recalls that their lodger, old Mrs Gurney (my maternal Grandmother, believe it or not, took in a lodger in her two-up-two-down house), had to go into the Workhouse. Many old ladies sewed 'burial money' into the hem of their skirts to avoid the indignity of a pauper's funeral

[84] See *Feminism and Family Planning in Victorian England, op cit.*

[85] *Birth Control and the Population Question in England 1877-1930, op cit,* p23.

[86] *Ibid.*

[87] In 1921, Dr C. V. Drysdale, President of the New Generation League (as the Malthusian League was later re-named), claimed: "...before the Knowlton trial...neither rich nor poor (most certainly not the latter) knew anything worth counting about contraceptive devices." (*The Malthusian*, November, 1921)

[88] (This average covers sixteen of the forty-one members of the NRBC (which sat from 1913-16) surveyed by Charles Edward Pell. (Pell, *The Law of Births and Deaths, Being a Study of the Variation in the Degree of Animal Fertility under the Influence of the Environment*, London, 1921, in Birth Control and the Population Question, p186.) Pell stated that the average fertility for the 188 women who told the NBRC before the war that they never practised birth control, was only 1.6 – fewer even than the 2.4 claimed by those who admitted using contraception.

[89] *Housewife*, Pelican Books, Middlesex, London, 1976.

[90] For discussion on modern feminist rejection of Freud's theories, see Hester Eisenstein, *Contemporary Feminist Thought*, Unwin Paperbacks, London, 1985.

[91] Published Dennis Dobson, London, 1979, p117.

[92] *ibid*

[93] Writing from Philadelphia, June 25th, 1745, in *Population, Evolution, and Birth Control: A collage of controversial ideas, op cit.*

[94] *Observations Concerning the Increase of Mankind*, 1755, in *Population, Evolution, and Birth Control, op cit.*

[95] Michael Schofield *Promiscuity*, Victor Gollancz Ltd., 1976, p33.

[96] *The Birth Controllers, op cit,* p34.

[97] *Elements of Social Science*, in *Birth Control, op cit,* p99.

[98] *ibid*

[99] Elizabeth Draper, *Birth Control in the Modern World*, Penguin, 1965, p93.

[100] *The Birth Controllers, op cit,* p76.

[101] *ibid* n34.

[102] *ibid* p180 n44.

[103] *ibid* pp102-3, n13-14.

[104] *Married Love*, in *ibid* p226 n10.

[105] *ibid* p238.

[106] *ibid* p103, n20.

[107] Ruth Picardie, in the *Independent* of 31.5.1996, writes of a 'History of Contraception' exhibition by Percy Skuy: "Skuy's favourite item in the collection is a cervical block: 'It looks like a little block, like a large dice about an inch square. It was given me by a doctor in New York City. It's made of wood. It was inserted into the vagina in the hope that one of the indentations would cover the cervix. A piece of string was attached to withdraw it. It was described as "an instrument of torture" because of its bulkiness and awkwardness.' Skuy interprets this as 'a story of motivation of creativity and probably equality'. His understanding of the fascinating social significance of his collection leaves a lot to be desired."

[108] Norman Himes, *Medical History of Contraception*, London, 1936, p94.

[109] From his *Memoires* p195.

[110] *The Birth Controllers, op cit,* p18.

[111] *ibid* p20.

[112] *ibid* p238.

[113] *ibid* p39.

[114] *Studies in Prolife Feminism*, Vol.1, No.3, Summer 1995.

[115] Glenda Cooper, "Long ago it was crocodile dung. Yesterday it was the Pill. Today, Persona", *Independent*, 28.4.97.

[116] *Birth Control, op cit,* p23.

[117] See *Medical History of Contraception*, p299.

[118] *The Birth Controllers, op cit,* pp24 & 32.

[119] *This Crowded Kingdom, op cit,* p40; Sheila Rowbotham, *A New World for Women*, Pluto Press, London, 1977, p22.

[120] M. Potts & P. Selman, *Society and Fertility*, 1979, p290.

[121] Sheila Rowbotham & Jeffrey Weeks, *Socialism and the New Life: the Personal and Sexual Politics of Edward Carpenter and Havelock Ellis*, Pluto Press, London, 1977, p14.

[122] Clive Wood & Beryl Suitters, *The Fight for Acceptance: A History of Contraception*, Medical & Technical Publishing Co. Ltd., 1970, p41.

[123] *This Crowded Kingdom, op cit,* p40.

[124] *Socialism and the New Life, op cit,* p17.

[125] Sheila Rowbotham, *Hidden From History: 300 years of Women's Oppression and the Fight Against It*, *Pluto Press*, 1973, pp74-75.

[126] *Feminism and Family Planning in Victorian England, op cit,* p91.

[127] *The Fight for Acceptance: A History of Contraception, op cit,* p139.

[128] *The Birth Controllers, op cit,* p161.

[129] Dr Halliday Sutherland, *Laws of Life*, Sheed & Ward, London, 1936, pp21-22.

[130] *The Birth Controllers, op cit,* p161.

[131] *ibid* p162.

[132] *Population, Evolution and Birth Control, op cit,* p199.

[133] In the event, he did not. *ibid*.

[134] *Laws of Life, op cit,* p22.

[135] *The Birth Controllers, op cit,* p164.

[136] The Malthusian League's first objective was to agitate for the abolition of all penalties on public debate of the 'population question'. (*The Birth Controllers,* p173)

[137] *Laws of Life, op cit,* p25.

[138] *The Birth Controllers, op cit,* p99.

[139] *ibid*

[140] *The Fight for Acceptance: A History of Contraception, op cit,* p107.

[141] *Birth Control in the Modern World, op cit,* p80.

[142] *The Fight for Acceptance: A History of Contraception, op cit,* p139.

[143] *Birth Control in the Modern World, op cit,* p80.

[144] *ibid*

[145] *The Fight for Acceptance: A History of Contraception, op cit,* p138.

[146] *ibid* p139.

[147] *The Fight for Acceptance: A History of Contraception, op cit*, pp138-9.

[148] *Birth Control in the Modern World, op cit*, p80.

[149] *Medical History of Contraception, op cit*, pp248-9.

[150] *Medical History of Contraception, op cit*, p249.

[151] *ibid*

[152] *Birth Control and the Population Question in England 1877-1930, op cit*, p112.

[153] *The Birth Controllers, op cit*, p307.

[154] *Medical History of Contraception, op cit*, p243.

[155] *Feminism and Family Planning in Victorian England, op cit*, p91.

[156] *Medical History of Contraception, op cit*, p249.

[157] *ibid*

[158] The proscribed times for intercourse, laid down in *Leviticus*, seem to ensure that intercourse would take place soon after a woman's period, which is indeed the most fertile time. (*Control of Life, op cit,* p233) Interestingly, the Bible is not mentioned in Elizabeth Draper's history of 'natural methods' of birth control in *Birth Control in the Modern World.*

[159] According to Himes (*Medical History of Contraception,* p82) Charles Knowlton "expressed doubts [about the reliability of coitus *interruptus*] for it had become evident that there were many unplanned pregnancies even when this method was most scrupulously carried out."(!)

[160] *Laws of Population, op cit*, pp21-2, in *Medical History of Contraception, op cit*, p246.

[161] *The Birth Controllers, op cit*, p110.

[162] G. K. Chesterton, *Eugenics and Other Evils*, Cassell & Co. Ltd., 1922.

[163] *Birth Control and the Population Question in England 1877-1930, op cit*, p60.

[164] *Elements of Social Science*, p366, in *Birth Control, op cit*, p122.

[165] *Elements of Social Science, op cit*, p353, in *ibid* p121.

[166] Essays in Medical Sociology, in *ibid* pp99-100.

[167] *The Birth Controllers, op cit*, pp74-5

[168] *Birth Control and the Population Question in England 1877-1930, op cit*, p112.

[169] Routh, *Moral and Physical Evils* pp11-13, in *Birth Control and the Population Question in England 1877-1930*, p113; see also *The Fight for Acceptance: A History of Contraception*, pp143-4.

[170] *Birth Control and the Population Question in England 1877-1930, op cit*, p128.

[171] *Birth Control, op cit*, p99.

[172] *Queen* v. *Bradlaugh and Besant*, pp107-109, in *Birth Control and the Population Question in England 1877-1930, op cit*, p60; see also Besant, *Laws of Population*, pp28-29.

[173] *Malthusian*, Feb 1889, pp1-2, in *Birth Control and the Population Question in England 1877-1930*, p91.

[174] *Physical, Sexual and Natural Religion*, in *The Birth Controllers*, p112.

[175] *Elements of Social Science, op cit*, p162, in *Birth Control*, p122.

[176] Letter, *New Generation*, November 1923, p133.

[177] *The Birth Controllers, op cit*, pp111-2.

[178] *Laws of Population, op cit*, p34, in *Medical History of Contraception*, p249.

[179] *Wife's Handbook*, published in the 1880s, in *ibid* p252.

[180] *The Birth Controllers, op cit,* p238.

[181] Dunlop to Stopes, 15 November 1917, Stopes Papers, Add. MS. 58564, in *Birth Control and the Population Question in England 1877-1930,* pp128-129.

[182] ibid

Chapter Two

EXPERIMENTING ON THE POOR

Marie Stopes, her trials, tribulations and triumphs; useless and dangerous methods; abortion and birth control.

The famous libel action brought by Marie Stopes against Dr Halliday Sutherland and his publishers in 1923 was treated as a *cause célèbre*. Stopes saw herself, not as the protagonist, but a victim of the Catholic Church.[1] The case has since been viewed as a triumph of publicity for birth control - with Marie, of course, as heroine.

Briefly, Stopes issued a writ for libel against a Catholic convert, Dr Sutherland. In his book *Birth Control*, under the heading, "Exposing the Poor to Experiment", Sutherland stated: "...the ordinary decent instincts of the poor [are] against these practices [birth control], and indeed they have used them less than any other class. But, owing to their poverty, lack of learning, and helplessness, the poor are the natural victims of those who seek to make experiments on their fellows. In the midst of a London slum a woman, who is a doctor of German philosophy (Munich), has opened a Birth Control Clinic, where working women are instructed in a method of contraception described by Professor McIlroy[2] as 'the most harmful method of which I have had experience.'"[3]

The verdict was confusing. The jury found that, though the words used were defamatory, they were true in substance and fact. However, they were not considered fair comment, and damages of £100 were awarded to Stopes.[4] Sutherland won on appeal. The case lasted two and a half years, and cost the defendants £10,000, which was raised by the Catholics of England, Scotland, Ireland and Wales.[5]

Seen in retrospect, the 'libel' in question should have been small provocation to someone of Stopes' standing. It could easily have been treated as fair criticism, or overlooked as the ramblings of a partisan, Catholic anti-birth control campaigner. But Stopes could not stand criticism, fair or unfair.[6] Worst of all, Sutherland's book exposed the hollowness of her claim that she wished to help the poor, and he used political, and economic, as well as religious and philosophical arguments to do so.

She was sensitive to reminders that she was not a medical doctor. Though she prescribed contraceptives with great authority,[7] she was not a doctor of medicine, but of Philosophy, having gained her Ph.D in Botany with Honours at Munich University.[8] Sutherland's medical credentials[9] must have grated appallingly on her ego.

In her first issue of *Birth Control News*, Stopes' review of Sutherland's book stated that it would "...impose only on those who are more ignorant than he is. It is nicely calculated to encourage the biased in their prejudices, for now, when speaking against birth control, they can say 'A doctor says so!' They will probably forget he is a Roman Catholic doctor."[10] She claimed the book's "omissions" were "quite as remarkable as its lies" and that columns could be filled "in illustration of this". However, the columns remained unfilled. "Space" she claimed, was "too valuable".[11]

Stopes knew of the great triumph attributed to Bradlaugh and Besant; the publicity of their trial was credited within the birth control movement (and without)[12] for the drop in the birth rate. Despite her previous connections and work with the Malthusians,[13] Stopes criticised Bradlaugh and Besant,[14] and abruptly severed her connections with the League.[15]

It is possible that she envied their success, and wanted to blot out their reputation for 'saving the world from people'. While correctly realising that the dramatic fall in the birth rate had in fact been coincidental to the trial, she began to see this fanatical handful of 'priests' with their grim Malthusian gospel as a stumbling block to the popular spread of birth control.

They may indeed have succeeded in drawing attention to their beliefs, but since those beliefs, when scrutinised, were found to be deeply unattractive, the publicity simply backfired. In truth, Stopes used the Malthusians to hitch a ride on the birth control bandwagon, but once safely aboard, typically, she seized the reins. With her sensational court case, she used their methods to finish the task they had begun, and so consolidated her place in history.

The irony was that despite their efforts, Bradlaugh, Besant, and the Malthusian League had failed to lower the birth rate of the poor. The League had even tried to convert the poor by going from house to house: "They would descend on working class areas for systematic house-to-house canvassing. They would thrust tracts and leaflets into the hands of the women who came to the doors and give verbal advice to all who listened."

Despite feeling they were "well-received by the poor" their efforts did not bear fruit. Neither could they find women 'missionaries' to do this work.[16] T. Owen Bonser, a League member and former fellow of Clare College, Cambridge, used to go on long summer walking tours, "talking to the peasantry and distributing Malthusian leaflets en route". Bonsor found that the poor could not pronounce the name of the League, calling it "Methusalem" - possibly a peasant's joke that Bonser failed to grasp.

Stopes, like the Malthusians, aimed her propaganda at the whole of society, but with a crucial difference: she wanted the better off to have more children, and the poor, fewer. Her exhortations were aimed at the rich; her birth control clinics were aimed at the poor. No one, it seemed, could force the rich to have more children; but they could try to prevent the poor having quite so many, or, ideally, none at all.

To encourage the middle classes to have more children, she fell back on flowery language, romanticised sex, and the joys of motherhood:

"Welling up in her are the wonderful tides, scented and enriched by the myriad experiences of the human race from its ancient days of leisure and flower-wreathed love-making, urging her to transports and self-expressions, were the man but ready to take the first step in the initiative or to recognise and welcome it in her." [17]

For the poor, however, she advocated contraceptives or sterilisation.[18] Unfortunately for Stopes - in common with others in the birth control movement - she was not an expert in birth control techniques. To working-class wives she recommended - if they could not afford two or three shillings for a rubber pessary - a sponge filled with soap powder, or a soluble quinine pessary.[19]

Stopes rejected criticism or differing opinions from colleagues, especially from doctors, whose knowledge of birth control she considered inferior, boasting: "I teach doctors."[20] Unlike some of her more pragmatic colleagues, however, who realised that people would simply stop using bad methods of birth control unless something more effective was developed, Stopes saw every doubt as a betrayal of herself and her perceived leadership of the modern birth control movement.[21]

The birth control methods advocated by early campaigners were ineffective, or dangerous, or both. The methods used by Stopes and fellow birth controllers in their clinics were not much better. Every method but the Dutch cap[22] was suspect, according to Stopes. She even recommended in 'Wise Parenthood' that rubber caps, together with quinine pessaries, be purchased from a chemist and self-fitted. Although she claimed to believe, with others, in the health-giving properties of semen to women,[23] it is hard to see how any health benefits could survive the quinine pessary.

Halliday Sutherland highlighted medical fears by referring to the check pessary acting as a contraceptive only "when it dams back the natural secretions of the womb. Consequently unless fitted by an expert and frequently removed under conditions of surgical cleanliness, the check pessary becomes a most dangerous and filthy appliance." He attributed its ineffectiveness to the difficulty of fitting the appliance even by a "skilled gynaecologist". He further revealed: "During the birth control libel action, a medical supporter of contraceptives stated that the check pessary had failed to prevent pregnancy in twenty-five out of twenty-nine cases in which it was tried."[24]

The birth controllers' need to portray the movement as respectable ruled out condoms, though they were advertised.[25] Despite their claims of a monopoly of knowledge on birth control, more research was plainly needed - especially into a more effective spermicide - in order to allay the fears of the medical profession.[26] So in 1927, the Birth Control Investigation Committee was 'born'. But it was necessary to test every new technique to allay well-founded medical suspicions that the methods advocated by birth controllers were unreliable.[27] Who better to test them on, than willing volunteers, who would surely flock to the clinics to avail themselves of what had formerly been reserved for their more fortunate sisters?

The trouble was, the willing volunteers were few in number. Many excuses were found for the poor's lack of eagerness for birth control. Poor women were too shy, it was alleged. They were frightened of entering the clinics. And of course, they were at the mercy of their brutal husbands. [28]

Many tactics were tried. First nurses were used, to reassure the 'patients'.[29] Then doctors were used, to reassure the medical profession. Then female doctors[30] - again, to reassure the 'patients'. Stopes' clinic (originally to be named 'The Humphrey Birth Control Clinic', after Marie's husband) was opened in Holloway, North London, as 'The Mother's Clinic'. It struck the right note. According to June Rose, "patients" were told that the Clinic was "'For Beauty' as well as for birth control; mothers would be considered not only as the producers of mere babies, but the creators of splendid babies." [31]

Perhaps the discovery that poor mothers actually cared what happened to their children, and wanted to keep them healthy, led to the emphasis on integrated mother and baby care. Ironically, it was to be utilised to try to prevent poor women from having children.

The Walworth Clinic, opened by the Drysdales in 1921, differed from Stopes' Holloway clinic, which opened eight months after, in that every woman was seen by a medical practitioner. The response was at first "very poor". (Fryer alleges shyness, despite the fact that the words 'birth control' were deliberately omitted from the clinic's name). Only two women attended in the whole of November 1921.

But by January 1923, it was said that attendance was up to 258, and that Dr Haire often saw "forty patients in a single afternoon" - certainly an amazing through-put. A sewing class and "little homely Birth Control talks" were given. But by July 1923, Fryer says that shortage of funds "compelled the abandonment of the ante-natal and baby clinics". From then on, it was to be birth control, and birth control only.[32]

In 1924 the campaigners, realising that progress could not be achieved through a handful of private clinics which were not popular with the women they were intended to reach, launched a political crusade to force local authorities to give out birth control 'advice' through their mother and baby clinics. In 1930, the Ministry of Health, responding to the pressure, quietly acquiesced.[33]

Margaret Pyke, Secretary of the National Birth Control Council (NBCC), described how clinic workers built on the foundations laid by the political campaigners. In 1932, she revealed, the Plymouth Medical Officer of Health, Dr A T Nankivell, suggested: "...he would lend us the premises of one of his Maternity and Child Welfare Centres and we would run a clinic. We could also have the help of one of the doctors on his staff who was keen to do this work.

So we formed a branch...in Plymouth, Lady Astor gave us £100, the Ministry of Health saw no objection."[34]

As for Stopes, her efforts to build up the popular image she craved as the lady bountiful of the birth control movement, included admiring pieces about herself in the Society for Constructive Birth Control's monthly magazine – pieces which Germaine Greer suspects were written either by her, or her compliant husband Humphrey.[35] As Stopes' biographer June Rose states: "...although the publicity exaggerated the clinic's progress the records did not. Despite claims that patients poured in, during the first year a timid trickle of three women a day on average rang the bell at No. 61."[36]

Rose says that even this was a "significant advance", given the prejudice with which birth control had to contend, but to Stopes, the need to be successful was vital. And as far as she was concerned, a client who never returned was a satisfied client, not one who had given up through contraceptive failure.[37]

Failure was foreign to Marie Stopes, even though others were more cautious: "Despite her husband's hesitant warnings that she needed to be careful not to inflate the number of patients who visited the clinic and overstate her successes, Stopes' claim of failure rates of between 0.52 and 2.5 percent in anywhere from 5,000 to 10,000 cases, was met with great scepticism, particularly when it was learned that she counted as a success any woman who did not return to the clinic or did not complain."[38]

Doctors were increasingly dependent on the new Birth Control Investigation Committee, and clinics' own reports, which assured them that most of the failures could be traced directly to human error or negligence rather than to a particular contraceptive.[39]

To a relentless self-publicist like Marie Stopes, the *Stopes v. Sutherland* libel action must have seemed a good way to drum up business, besides enshrining her reputation as leader of the burgeoning birth control movement. Unfortunately for her, facts got in the way. The jury found that she really *had* been experimenting on the poor. Besides recommending vaseline and soap powder[40] for poor women who wished to avoid children, the incident of Dr Norman Haire and the 'gold pin' was enough to encourage doubts of Stopes' veracity.

Damning evidence was given at the libel trial of a case where Stopes had referred two patients to Dr Norman Haire, asking him to insert a 'gold pin', (an intrauterine device). When he did not comply, having already investigated the device at her request, and found it could cause septic abortion and pelvic infection, she wrote: "I should like very much for you, if you do not mind, to take on two or three cases, which you should watch carefully, and if these yielded unsatisfactory results we would then drop it."[41]

Any lingering doubts about Stopes' readiness to experiment on the poor are laid to rest by her own 1925 report, which clearly states the aims behind the

Mothers' Clinic for Constructive Birth Control. They were "to obtain first-hand facts about contraception in practice".[42]

Doubtless, it was felt by others in the birth control movement that Stopes was not only giving out dangerous 'advice' - nothing new - she was also being *seen* to give out dangerous advice. So, despite his support for her aims, Haire gave evidence against her.[43] Soloway describes Haire as "a reluctant defense witness who, however much he admired her objectives, questioned some of her contraceptive recommendations."[44]

Where birth control history is concerned, the facts must never be allowed to get in the way of a good story, and Marie Stopes remains perhaps the best-known name associated with the birth control campaign in this country. However, her greatest triumph was not in dispensing birth control, but in converting a movement hostile to women, into a women's' crusade. She converted a libertarian male campaign for sex without babies, into a women's campaign for better motherhood and sexual fulfilment, thus outflanking the feminists who argued that birth control was another weapon against women. Women might continue to be oppressed, but Marie Stopes could help them to enjoy the manacles.

She overrode the insulting Malthusian idea that the poor were responsible for their own poverty, insisting that they could be responsible for their own happiness. She took the politics of birth control and (to abuse the *lingua franca* of modern feminism), she succeeding in making the political personal.

Failure was not a deterrent to Stopes who, despite evidence to the contrary, still claimed success.[45] Others were more sanguine, calling for scientific investigation into more reliable methods of birth control.[46] But one natural method that *was* becoming more reliable was not included in their investigations.

New discoveries were being made concerning the 'safe period', making it more accurate.[47] Ironically, the birth control campaign now started to warn against it as unreliable, though previously, they had advocated it alongside equally dubious methods.[48] So why did not the campaigners advocate something which, being completely free, would be more likely to be used by the section of society which they targeted – the poor?

Birth Control and Abortion

As we have noted, the dangers of contraception had always been seen as incidental by birth controllers, who frankly acknowledged that they needed to experiment on the poor, while at the same time dismissing lurid accusations of anti-birth control doctors as laughable.[49] However, a modern-day physician who has worked in family planning, Dr Ellen Grant, reveals: "An interesting study found a link with ovarian cancer and talcum powder, which can back-track through the womb along the tubes and reach the ovaries, where it acts as an irritant like asbestos. Thirty years ago it was the custom to tell women to keep their caps dry by covering them in talcum powder" [50]

The long-term effects of contraception were of little concern to the majority of birth controllers. They were indifferent, too, to the immediate side effects of birth control, their only anxiety being that women might stop using contraception. They knew very little about fertility. Most importantly, they knew that the birth control methods they advocated were not totally reliable, but pressed on regardless. Did this determination to spread the use of birth control, despite its unreliability, actually lead to more abortions? For in giving the world the 'planned' pregnancy, the birth controllers also invented the unplanned pregnancy.

The history of the birth control campaign is full of stern condemnations of abortion. Soloway tells us: "From its earliest days the Malthusian League struggled to keep the two separate in the public's mind, condemning abortion as illegal, dangerous, and unnecessary."[51] On closer examination, this is not a condemnation at all. It merely points out that abortion is 'illegal' (obvious); 'dangerous' (also obvious); and 'unnecessary' (because there was such a thing as birth control).

The last word gives us a clue to the motivations of the Malthusians in 'condemning' abortion. They used it as a warning - of what would happen if people did not accept birth control. In similar vein C.V. Drysdale, in 1913, claimed that abortion was a failure of prevention; one was criminal, the other was not. (He meant the failure to *use* contraceptives, not the failure *of* contraceptives.)[52]

To those who considered birth control as an evil (probably the majority), abortion was portrayed as an even greater evil. To these objectors, the Malthusians promised, "termination of pregnancy would, like prostitution, become unnecessary and rare if the campaign for birth control succeeded". So much for what is described in the same paragraph as their "unwavering opposition to abortion". In truth, as Soloway goes on to say, "...the league insisted that it would be folly to waste energy and resources championing an imperfect remedy, which would only seem to validate the malicious charges the organization had refuted for decades".[53]

The story of the birth control campaign and the issue of abortion is a tangled one, as we will see. The Malthusian League, according to Olive Banks, condemned abortion as a "crime, the murder of the child in the womb".[54] In 1915, a Malthusian League memorandum made it clear that they were not prepared to consider the subject, following American birth controller Margaret Sanger's insistence in her pamphlet *Family Limitation* that abortion, though not to be considered as a method of birth control, should be done as early in the pregnancy as possible.[55]

Linda Gordon, in *Woman's Body, Woman's Right*, claims that Sanger, apparently influenced by the English sexologist Havelock Ellis, "defended a women's rights to an abortion, something she was never to do at any later time".[56] Elasah Drogin writes that Ellis advised Sanger to moderate her stance on abortion – of which she approved – because it would be more productive to

49

her cause to stick to one issue: birth control. So she set out to use abortion to enhance the respectability of birth control – birth control, she claimed, would put an end to abortion.[57]

In 1914, with a few hundred dollars from Edward Bond Foote, Sanger printed a pamphlet *Family Limitation*, containing information regarding birth control, but could not mail her journal *Woman Rebel*, containing the information, because the authorities deemed it obscene. According to Gordon, the pamphlet "recommended and explained a variety of contraceptives - douches, condoms, pessaries, sponges and vaginal suppositories". More to the point, it also "gave a suggestion for an abortifacient".[58] She was prosecuted in 1915, and fled the country. She later criticised the Soviet Union for restricting legal abortion and birth control in the 1930s, comparing Mussolini, Stalin and Hitler to the Catholic Church for encouraging births.[59]

Despite evidence that she thought both birth control *and* abortion were necessary to control fertility, Sanger claimed it was as a result of attending a fatal self-abortion that she had become involved in the birth control campaign.[60] Sanger had no hesitation in using the tragedy of abortion deaths to underline the consequences of not giving poor women birth control.

Despite alleged qualms about abortion, the Malthusian League was happy to support the English publishers of Sanger's Family *Limitation*, when the publishers were prosecuted for obscenity for producing its revised 1923 edition. The pamphlet, according to Lord Amberley (Bertrand Russell's elder brother), justified abortion, as he advised Marie Stopes.[61] Stopes subsequently declined to support the defendants, giving this as her reason.[62] Just to confuse matters further, the publisher, Rose Witcop, in her introduction to the Sanger pamphlet, alleges that birth control will mean "fewer complaints due to abortion".[63]

Perhaps Sanger, in the original pamphlet, was following the example of birth controller Richard Carlile, who wrote his ironically-titled *Every Woman's Book* in the early nineteenth century to counteract the evil of infanticide and abortion, while including two methods of abortion in it![64]

The birth controllers appeared ready to change their story according to the audience, and whether there was a chance of prosecution. They were not averse to prosecution, but on the contrary, carefully planned and executed their 'crimes' in order to challenge, and possibly change, the law. Like Sanger, they were prepared to test the temperature of public opinion on abortion, hastily withdrawing their toe if the water proved too hot. Far from responding to the public's need for birth control, they were constantly trying to push back the frontiers of social acceptability, testing the legality of their actions, rallying support to make every court case a *cause célèbre*, using the resultant publicity to spread birth control propaganda.

Their indifference to the evil of abortion, concentrating as they did on whether it was legal, or necessary,[65] and using tragic cases to promote contraception,[66] shows that their interest was not in the victims of abortion.

This is because, to the population controllers, abortion - or even infanticide - was not the greatest evil. We turn again to the stalwart of the Malthusian League, Dr C. R. Drysdale, who asserted that begetting such numbers as 20, 21, or 25 children was "...one of the greatest social crimes a man could commit".[67] To the Malthusian League, people (or overpopulation, or population growth) were the greatest evil. Consequently, they felt little sympathy for those who eased the problem by their own demise.

The methods advocated by the birth controllers - like abortion, which they hesitated to promote - were all 'imperfect remedies'. They must have led to many unplanned pregnancies. It is most unlikely that the campaigners could embrace birth control so wholeheartedly if they did not privately approve of - or at least were indifferent to - abortion. Norman Himes - himself a birth control advocate - suggests in his *Medical History of Contraception,* that the prosecution of Dr Allbutt's *Wife's Handbook* had a great deal to do with the fact that it contained advertisements for abortifacients.[68] The Malthusian League - consistent as ever - leapt to Allbutt's defence.[69]

Another instance of the Malthusians' blundering was the issue of breast feeding. By condemning it as a method of contraception,[70] Besant may have contributed to the decline of a practice vital for the health of poor babies, whose mortality rate was worsened as a result of insanitary bottle-feeding.[71] Her condemnation may also have contributed to the bad health of their mothers, who relied on breast-feeding to 'space' their children naturally.[72]

Of course, breast feeding to space children was no good to the ideal Malthusian family, which consisted of a couple who married young, produced two children, and then had no more for the rest of their natural lives. As late as 1965, birth control historian Elizabeth Draper warns about breast-feeding as a method of family planning.[73]

Besant, though she condemned abortion,[74] also cited medical "testimony" to show that it was sometimes "medically indicated", and therefore necessary. Draper confirms this, telling us: "Even Mrs Besant in the late nineteenth century advocated termination of pregnancy in medical cases."[75] It is likely that, in common with other birth controllers, Besant pitched her game to whoever was playing. For those who detested abortion, she could warn that abortion would increase if birth control were not widely adopted, while to those who already approved of birth control (and perhaps realised that it was faulty), she could admit to cautious approval of abortion.

Marie Stopes is on record as detesting abortion.[76] She insisted that her clinic workers swear an oath not to perform abortion "in any circumstances". She accused one lover, Avro Manhattan, of "murdering" an infant, after hearing that one of his woman friends had become pregnant and had had an abortion. She wrote in 1923 to the Director of Public Prosecutions regarding the Aldred case that abortion was "both criminal and harmful".[77] A genuine abhorrence may have stemmed from the stillbirth of her first child. But Stopes also quietly referred women for abortion - or "evacuation of the uterus", as she termed it - if she (not a medical doctor, as we have seen) deemed it necessary.[78]

We have already seen how Stopes experimented on 'patients' with the abortifacient gold pin. She had mentioned it several times in her books, but always, according to biographer Ruth Hall, with the "proviso that it must be fitted by a doctor, and that its effects were not fully known." Despite this, as Hall relates, only a month after her clinic opened, Stopes' eagerness led her to ask the Surgical Manufacturing Company to make to her specifications "a small simple pin of flexible vulcanite or celluloid medicated so as to be suitable for internal use."[79]

The willingness of the birth control campaign to experiment continued, unabated by occasional disasters. Dr Alan Guttmacher, writing the preface to *Medical History of Contraception*,[80] relates how Dr Ernst Grafenberg's 'silver ring', introduced in 1929, had attracted "many qualified opponents". He tells how the abortifacient device caused "occasional erosion through the walls of the uterus" and mentioned the "inflammation and bleeding which it sometimes caused".

The fate of the human guinea pigs concerned is not recorded. Nevertheless, researchers continued to experiment with such devices, using a variety of materials. In relating the story of these experiments (including the notorious Dalkon Shield), and the obfuscation employed to disguise their real effects, Germaine Greer makes clear that such devices act as abortifacients.[81]

Warnings about abortion from population controllers, while muddying the historical waters of the birth control campaign, at least give us a clue to public opinion on an important issue. The fact that they found it necessary to spice their exhortations to use birth control, with warnings of increased abortions, leads us to the inevitable conclusion that the public found abortion abhorrent - an abhorrence that dwarfed even their distaste for birth control.

NOTES

[1] Germaine Greer, *Sex and Destiny*, *op cit*, p311.

[2] Louise McIlroy, a leading birth control opponent who, however (according to Stopes, in Keith Briant's biography), fitted her with a rubber cap when she visited McIlroy at the Royal Free Hospital disguised as a "work-grimed charwoman". (*The Birth Controllers, p231.*)

[3] Proceedings of the Medico-Legal Society, July 7th, 1921, in Halliday Sutherland MD (Edinburgh), Birth *Control: A Statement of Christian Doctrine against the Neo-Malthusians*, Harding & More Ltd, 1922, pp101-2

[4] See *Laws of Life*, Chapter 2; also Ruth Hall, *Marie Stopes: a biography*, Andre Deutsch, 1977, Chapter13.

[5] *Laws of Life, op cit.*

[6] *Sex and Destiny, op cit*, p311.

[7] To an enquirer, she responded: "I do not practice medicine in the ordinary way but I have had forced upon myself an unofficial consultation sort of practice on sex, psychology and physiology." Occasionally she charged two or three guineas for an "unofficial consultation" by post.

(CMAC:PP/MCS:A.197, in June Rose, *Marie Stopes and the Sexual Revolution*, Faber & Faber, 1992, p119)

[8] *Marie Stopes and the Sexual Revolution, op cit*, p34

[9] See Chapter Five

[10] *Marie Stopes: a biography, op cit*, p207.

[11] *ibid*

[12] Ethel Elderton, a eugenic investigator, in common with other late Victorian and Edwardian birth rate investigators, blamed the Bradlaugh-Besant trial for the fall in the birth rate. In her *Report on the English Birthrate*, she claimed the Bradlaugh-Besant trial "legitimised the teaching of practical methods for the limitation of the family, and within thirty years that teaching has revolutionised the sexual habits of the English people". She also blamed them for causing the differential birth rate. (*Birth Control and the Population Question in England 1877-1930*, p53)

[13] *Birth Control and the Population Question in England 1877-1930, op cit*, p223.

[14] *The Workers' Dreadnought* (10.3.1923) criticised Stopes for supporting the prosecution of Bradlaugh and Besant, and later, Margaret Sanger and the Aldreds, "for a birth control propaganda which, in effect, is the same as her own". The jury in the *Stopes v Sutherland and Others* libel case had found the accusation to be true in substance and fact, that Stopes' literature was not less obscene than that for which Bradlaugh and Besant were found guilty. In other words, it was a case of the pot calling the kettle black. (*Laws of Life*, pp33-34)

[15] She suddenly 'discovered' their Atheism. (*Birth Control and the Population Question in England 1877-1930*, pp224-5)

[16] Besant's successor as Secretary, William Hammond Reynolds, advertised in 1889 for a "lady Malthusian missionary to work from house to house" - without success. (*The Malthusian*, December 1889, in *The Birth Controllers*, pp173-174)

[17] *Married Love*, p20

[18] See *Marie Stopes and the Sexual Revolution*; also *Marie Stopes: a biography*

[19] *Letter to Working Mothers*, p5, in *Birth Control and the Population Question in England 1877-1930*, p215.

[20] See *Birth Control and the Population Question in England 1877-1930*, pp268-9, for her disagreements with Norman Haire on methods of birth control and his testimony in the libel case.

[21] *Birth Control and the Population Question in England 1877-1930, op cit*, pp268-9

[22] See *Sex and Destiny*, p315, for Stopes' insistence on the Dutch cap in preference to the smaller cervical cap; also *Birth Control and the Population Question in England 1877-1930*, p214

[23] *Birth Control and the Population Question in England 1877-1930, op cit*, p314

[24] *Laws of Life, op cit*, p38

[25] The 'Malthusian' carried advertisements for 'rubber goods'; so did Sanger's pamphlet *Family Limitation*.

[26] See *Birth Control and the Population Question in England 1877-1930*, Chapter12 'The Medical Profession'.

[27] In his ironically-titled *Wife's Handbook* (1887 edition), Dr Allbutt enthused, regarding Rendell's soluble pessaries: "It is but right to say that these pessaries are at present only on trial. Time will show whether they can be relied upon to prevent conception. My opinion is that they will do all their inventor claims for them". (*Medical History of Contraception*, p253)

[28] According to Katherine Gamgee "...most of the suffering of our working-class women arises from the unrestrained licence and want of self-control of their husbands..." ('Public Health',

October 1925, in *Birth Control and the Population Question in England 1877-1930*, p272; see also *The Fight for Family Planning*, Chapter 1.

[29] Margaret Sanger advised the Drysdales to establish a clinic staffed with nurses, as she had seen in Holland. (*Birth Control and the Population Question in England 1877-1930*, p189)

[30] See *Birth Control and the Population Question in England 1877-1930*, Chapter 9, for Dr Norman Haire's replacement at the Malthusian Walworth Clinic by an advisory medical council of female physicians and a woman supervisor.

[31] *Marie Stopes and the Sexual Revolution, op cit*, p145

[32] *The Birth Controllers, op cit*, pp251-2

[33] *The Birth Controllers*, Chapter 22; also *The Fight for Family Planning*, Chapter 5

[34] M. Pyke, *Family Planning: An Assessment, Eugenics Review*, LV, 2 (1963), in *The Fight for Family Planning,*, p51

[35] *Sex and Destiny, op cit*, p315

[36] *Marie Stopes and the Sexual Revolution, op cit*, p145

[37] For discussion of Stopes', and others', exaggerated claims of success, see *Birth Control and the Population Question in England 1877-1930*, Chapter 12.

[38] Marie Stopes, *The First Five Thousand*, in *Marie Stopes, Eugenics and the The English Birth Control Movement*, ed. Robert A. Peel, The Galton Institute, 1997, p64

[39] *Birth Control and the Population Question in England 1877-1930, op cit*, p277

[40] "...a small wet sponge whose pores were filled with powdered soap, or a pad of cotton wool smeared with vaseline". (M. Stopes, *Wise Parenthood*, 1918, in *The Birth Controllers*, p226)

[41] Muriel Box, *The Trial of Marie Stopes*, London, 1967, pp292-4, in *Sex and Destiny* p315; see also *Birth Control and the Population Question in England 1877-1930*, pp268-9

[42] *The First Five Thousand*, in *The Fight for Family Planning*, p12

[43] Norman Haire - the doctor originally in charge of the Malthusian League's Walworth Road clinic in London - was subpoenaed by the defence in the Stopes *v* Sutherland libel trial. He gave evidence against Marie reluctantly. (*Marie Stopes: a biography*, pp232-3)

[44] Box, *Trial of Marie Stopes*, in *Birth Control and the Population Question in England 1877-1930*, p268

[45] See *Marie Stopes, Eugenics and The English Birth Control Movement, op cit*

[46] See *Birth Control and the Population Question in England 1877-1930*, Chapter12

[47] In Chapter 4 of his 1936 book *Laws of Life* (Sheed & Ward), Halliday Sutherland explains previous mistakes made in calculating the 'safe period'. He provides a perpetual calendar to enable any woman to calculate her own 'safe period', using the discoveries of Ogino and Knaus, the former in Japan, in 1930, and the latter in Austria in 1931, independently of each other. Briefly, they discovered that the timing of menstruation depended on the time of ovulation, and that it was possible to calculate back (providing the length of the cycle was known) to the probable time of ovulation. They also took into account the life of a sperm being longer than that of an egg, necessitating a longer period of abstinence. Sutherland also points out that Mosaic Law was cognisant of the fertile period. See also *The Fight for Acceptance: A History of Contraception*, p119, for Pouchet's discoveries regarding ovulation in the nineteenth century.

[48] It is interesting to note that, though still insisting on *douching*, Sanger appears to have revised her ideas on its efficacy as a birth control method, and claims it is for reasons of "hygiene", not contraception.(*Family Limitation*, 1925 edition).

[49] See references to medical objections, *op cit*.

[50] *Sexual Chemistry: Understanding Our Hormones, the Pill and HRT*, Cedar, 1994, p53

[51] *Birth Control and the Population Question in England 1877-1930, op cit,* p117

[52] Drysdale, *Small Family System,* pp8-9, in *Birth Control and the Population Question in England 1877-1930,* p118

[53] Malthusian League, Fortieth Annual Report; also 'Malthusian', November 1916 and February 1917, in *Birth Control and the Population Question in England 1877-1930,* p118

[54] Citing Rosanna Ledbetter's *A History of the Malthusian League 1877-1927,* Columbus, Ohio State University Press, 1976, in *Faces of Feminism,* p191; see also *The Birth Controllers,* p239 and *Birth Control in the Modern World,* p320.

[55] 'Memorandum Concerning the Prosecution of Mrs Margaret H. Sanger of New York, USA, for Her Advocacy of Birth Control and Her Issue of a Pamphlet Entitled "Family Limitation" Describing Various Methods of Restricting Families', the International Neo-Malthusian Bureau of Correspondence and Defence (London, 1915), in *Birth Control and the Population Question in England 1877-1930,* p343

[56] *Woman's Body, Woman's Right: Birth Control in America,* Penguin revised ed., 1990, p219

[57] Elasah Drogin, T.O.P., *Margaret Sanger: Father of Modern Society,* p.69, CUL Publications, 1980. The author is noted as a Jewish convert to Catholicism, living in a Dominican Third Order Lay Community in California. At time of writing, she was President of Catholics United for Life, and had spoken frequently in public and in the media about her own abortion, and the genocidal effects of abortion and sterilisation.

[58] Sanger, *My Fight for Birth Control,* p.87; Sanger Diary, 1914, in Sanger Papers, Library of Congress. ????> *Autobiography,* M. Sanger, W W Norton, New York, 1938, pp108-17, > is this full name of Sanger's Diary?? in *Woman's Body, Woman's Right,* p219

[59] Sanger to P B P Huse, January 2, 1940, in Sanger, Sophia Smith collection, Smith College, in *Woman's Body, Woman's Right,* p316

[60] Alice Jenkins, *Law for the Rich,* Charles Skilton Ltd., London, 1964

[61] E. Russell to Stopes, 18.1.23, in *Birth Control and the Population Question in England 1877-1930,* p230

[62] Muriel Box, *The Trial of Marie Stopes,* p294, in *Marie Stopes: a biography,* p210

[63] *ibid* p4

[64] One by inserting instruments such as knitting needles into the womb, the other by ingesting ergot of rye, savine and "violent purgatives". (*Every Woman's Book; or What is Love? Containing Most Important Instructions for the Prudent Regulation of the Principle of Love and the Number of A Family,* in *Sex and Destiny,* p297)

[65] In his foreword to *Medical History of Contraception,* R. L. Dickinson calls abortion and infanticide an "extravagant waste", while on p281, E. B. Foote (Dr Edward Bond Foote, American physician, whose views on contraception were published in 'Critic and Guide' in 1910) is recorded as saying that under all circumstances "contraception is preferable to abortion, and should as far as possible be substituted for it".

[66] Knowlton claimed, in *Fruits of Philosophy,* that birth control would reduce abortion and infanticide, displaying a dismal lack of insight into the causes of such evils – see *The Birth Controllers,* p103

[67] In evidence given at the Bradlaugh and Besant trial, *The Birth Controllers,* p163

[68] Himes states: "Allbutt liked to make it appear that his sole offence had been to publish a hygienic pamphlet, allegedly indecent, *at a low price.* But the case was not so simple as this. ...Allbutt was diffusing medical knowledge in a form generally not approved by physicians - the issuance of popular medical treatises. Trademarked articles of various kinds were recommended to the general public. Though the edition of the 'Wife's Handbook' of 1886 (third) contained

advertisements of contraceptive supplies, and though Allbutt rigorously condemned abortion in his pamphlet, the brochure in which he defended himself against treatment by the General Medical Council contained two advertisements of retail distributors of abortifacient pills."(*Medical History of Contraception,* p255)

[69] *Medical History of Contraception, op cit*

[70] *Laws of Population, op cit*

[71] See Elizabeth Roberts, *A Woman's Place: An Oral History of Working-class Women 1890-1940,* Basil Blackwell, 1985, for a description of the long tube bottles still in use in 1911, "with a couple of feet of rubber tubing between bottle and teat, [which] would be difficult to sterilise even today, and must have been a paradise for germs before the first world war". (p166) In 1911, Preston Health Visitors reported on 111 babies who had died of diarrhoea, only eight of whom were breast-fed, six partly breast-fed, and ninety-six bottle-fed. (Medical Officer of Health for Preston, 'Annual Report', 1911 *ibid*)

[72] "Throughout the world as a whole, more births are prevented by lactation than all other forms of contraception put together...The more unfavourable the environment, the more infant survival and birth spacing both become dependent on breast feeding." (R. V. Short, 'The evolution of human reproduction', *Proceedings of the Royal Society of London,* B, Vol. 195 (1976) p.17, in *Sex and Destiny,* p105)

[73] *Birth Control in the Modern World, op cit,* p88

[74] See *Medical History of Contraception, op cit,* p247.

[75] *Birth Control in the Modern World, op cit,* p106

[76] See *Marie Stopes: a biography,* p210; also *Marie Stopes and the Sexual Revolution,* p143.

[77] Box, *The Trial of Marie Stopes,* p294

[78] See *Marie Stopes: a biography, op cit*

[79] 12 April 1921, MCS to the Surgical Manufacturing Company. (British Library, Marie Stopes Collection)

[80] *op cit,* pp*xxvi - xxvii*

[81] *Sex and Destiny, op cit,* Chapter 7.

Chapter Three

A POPULAR MASS MOVEMENT?

The popularity of birth control; alternative methods; birth control and infanticide; the politics of birth control.

Chapter Two looked at the apparent success enjoyed by the birth control movement by the 1930s. This may lead us to believe that it was a popular mass movement. Books on birth control certainly sold well,[1] but so did anything relating to sex. Many copies would have been sold to the 'converted' i.e. other Malthusian groups, both in Britain and abroad.

Birth control appliances sold well, too. By the end of the nineteenth century, the Malthusian League claimed to be receiving two thousand requests per month for contraceptive appliances, advertisements for which filled their monthly magazine.[2] Whether they were sold to Malthusians, chemists, or ordinary members of the public, newly-converted to birth control - or less reputable people interested in the abortifacient uses of, for example, syringes – is not clear. It is unlikely that they were purchased or used by the poor.

Birth control historians claim that it became a respectable topic of conversation. Fryer claims that contraceptive knowledge and practice was widespread,[3] and that commentators on population decline blamed, amongst other things, the growth of towns for "facilitating both the spread of information over garden walls and in factories…"[4] Indeed, Potts and Selman claim that it was "thrown on to the breakfast tables of the English middle classes".[5]

But some, at least, objected to having unsolicited birth control literature 'thrown onto their breakfast tables', like the minister whose son-in-law received twelve advertisements for contraceptives a few days after the birth of his child.[6] The births, marriages – and even deaths - columns of newspapers were often used in this way to sell all manner of goods. It was not in the best possible taste, but taste has been historically lacking in the birth control campaign. More recently, a deputy editor of the *Nursing Times* related: "I can vividly recall the midwife who discharged me from hospital. As she said goodbye, she tried to press some condoms into my hand 'to keep you going until you get to a family planning clinic'. I could hardly walk at the time, let alone contemplate sex. And yes – she had read my notes."[7]

For some years in British hospitals, it has been customary to enquire into the contraceptive plans of new mothers, illustrating the fact that, far from waning, Malthusian obsessions have been officially taken on board, with the kind of brisk 'sensible shoes' attitude of which only the English are capable.

Yet despite the enthusiasm of their founders, and inflated claims of success, the first birth control clinics suffered severe lack of custom. And it was clear that the families of the poor – the main concern of the birth control movement - were still very large compared to middle- and upper class families.

Birth control historians try to solve this puzzle by dividing the population into 'people' and 'society'. Thus (according to Peter Fryer) though 'everyone' was using family limitation, the "prevailing social climate" was "too dense an obstacle".[8] Apparently, 'the people' wanted birth control, but 'society' would not let them have it.[9] And the Banks' contention that one of the causes of the falling birth rate in the late nineteenth century was the financial burden of having children,[10] cannot be applied to the poor, who were worst off, but had most children.

In the late nineteenth century, artificial birth control methods available were very unreliable, and more likely to result in pregnancy than prevent it. Condoms were mostly used for the prevention of disease by the man, rather than to prevent pregnancy. The business only really began to get into its stride with the vulcanisation of rubber, discovered by Goodyear and Hancock in the 1840s. Supplies were imported - mainly from Germany – until the 1930s.[11]

The main supplier, LRC Products, only began in 1915, when L.A. Jackson set up as a "wholesaler of chemists sundries", in one room behind a tobacconist's shop in the City of London, as an outlet for imported supplies of the contraceptive. However, the fact that any product was on sale did not necessarily mean that 'everyone' knew about it, and that those who did know, automatically went out to buy it, especially if it had no relevance to their beliefs or lifestyle. Many people may have been aware of ways of preventing conception, just as may have been aware of ways of charming warts.

After the First World War, attendance by working-class women at the first birth control clinics was low. Sometimes the methods failed, and they did not return. As C. P. Blacker, Secretary of the Eugenics Society later reported, though total attendance had risen substantially, there had been an absolute *decrease* in the numbers of working class women attending clinics.[12] Condom manufacture was hardly adequate to supply the needs of the whole country,[13] even if the whole country wanted them, though during 1917, they were distributed among troops by a government anxious about the scourge of sexually transmitted diseases.[14] This was to protect soldiers, not prevent births. In fact, it was partly out of concern for their wives and any children who might be born to them later. The danger to women and children from the sexual misbehaviour of men was an important theme of feminists. They were worried by ailing children and ill health and sterility suffered by women,[15] in stark contrast to the emphasis of modern feminism, which concentrates more on the right to engage freely in sex, than on the consequent dangers to women.

As far as the poor were concerned, who had enough to do to feed, clothe and house themselves on a pittance, condoms would have been expensive to purchase regularly. They could be unreliable - even taking into account the fact that women are fertile for only a few days a month - besides being aesthetically repellant to men (known colloquially as 'passion killers'), and insulting to their wives. Contraceptive use could also be what is known colloquially as a palaver, as Margaret Sanger shows in *Family Limitation*:

"The condom should be washed before and after putting it into the jar of alcohol and should be kept tightly corked. It is almost impossible to keep skin condoms satisfactorily if they are dried.... It is desirable to discard the condom after it has been used once unless with certain precautions. If it is to be used again care must be taken to wash the condom in an antiseptic solution before drying it and placing it away for further use. A weak solution of lysol is excellent for the rubber condom. The condom should be well lubricated with oil before penetration. It should always be tested for holes or breaks before using."[16]

While stressing that douching after sex could not be relied upon as a contraceptive, Sanger still gives instructions for douching 'recipes'.[17] Referring to it as a "cleanser", she goes into extraordinary detail, recommending: "If you have bathing conveniences, go as quickly as possible to the bathroom after the sexual act and prepare a douche. Lie down upon the back in the bath tub. Hang the filled douche bag high over the tub, and let the water flow freely into the vagina, to wash out the male sperm which was deposited during the act."[18] She also gives instructions for those without "bathroom conveniences": "a douche can be taken over the toilet, or when that is impossible" (perhaps because the 'convenience' was at the end of the garden, and therefore not very convenient) "it can be taken over a vessel in a squatting position".[19]

Those whose romantic inclinations survived the palaver of washing and drying condoms, or sprinting to the bathroom immediately after sex, would find the 'rubber shops' (where contraceptives were sold), tended to be found in big cities like London. They did most of their business by mail order, mainly because they were not seen as respectable places to be seen entering. In *A Woman's Place*, an oral history of working-class Lancashire women from 1890 to 1940, working class contributors confirm that birth control was not widely practised at all.[20] Other writers, with evidence just as scanty and vague, nevertheless deduce that birth control was widely practised, from the fact of the falling birth rate.[21]

The 'withdrawal method', or *coitus interruptus*, had been around for a very long time. It was certainly known about in Biblical times, since the story of Onan, who 'spilled his seed upon the ground', rather than risk impregnating his dead brother's widow.[22] Germaine Greer hypothesises that 'withdrawal' had been widely practised,[23] but it gradually lost ground to artificial contraception.[24]

With the advent of the birth control movement, there was a vested interest in promoting new, more 'reliable' methods, while warning against older 'unreliable' ones. The old methods, of course, cost nothing, did not need to be marketed, and made a profit for no one. They had the added advantage of not involving a third party in an intimate relationship. As one contributor to *A Woman's Place* remarked: "You couldn't get pills. We were on the bus and Harold knew the conductor and he asked Harold if we were married. He said, 'Don't forget, always get off the bus at South Shore, don't go all the way to Blackpool.'"[25] The method could be used to suit the couple's financial circumstances. Any bad effects (though certainly not as drastic as those alleged by the Malthusians), had to be balanced against what a couple thought they might gain from practising it.

If a woman was in ill health, a husband could practise abstinence, and sleeping apart was common in working-class households. Beds were shared with babies or children.[26] And there was breast feeding, as another correspondent pointed out: "Well, [breast feeding] was healthier and it was good for you as well. If it stopped you having another baby, it helped. It didn't stop you, but it helped. They said in those days that while you were feeding you couldn't conceive. Some did, but it did help. It was a good thing."[27]

Mary Wollstonecraft, author of *Vindication of the Rights of Woman*, and regarded as one of the earliest feminists, wrote in 1792: "For Nature has so wisely ordered things, that did women suckle their children, they would preserve their own health, and there would be such an interval between the birth of each child, that we should seldom see a houseful of babes."[28]

Evidence of these natural methods is bound to be patchy, since no records were kept,[29] and, of course, no sales were involved. Ironically, we have the ritual condemnations of the birth controllers to thank for bringing these methods to our attention, in addition to knowledge handed down. By the end of the Second World War, it is probable that many younger men knew of male contraceptive methods, but women were often ignorant of both male and female artificial methods.[30]

We must beware of drawing too many conclusions about the practice, or non-practice, of something so entirely personal in the lives of our forebears, when even visits to the lavatory were shrouded in polite euphemism. Our so-called sexually open society means virtual, not real, openness. It is a discourse conducted and regulated not by the public, but by professional entertainers and pundits. Computers, videos, books, magazines, and even TV talk shows or 'soaps' do not equate actual experience.

Even today, in the *real* world, sex is a private matter. There are very few people with whom we would discuss sexual practices and birth control methods – especially not at the bus stop, or in the supermarket. The situation of home and work place is, of course, a slightly different matter. But discussions with neighbours on these personal matters, conducted whilst raking the leaves, are probably no more than wishful thinking for those who see history as a foreign land, yet cannot believe that anything was ever 'done differently' there.

At the root of people's rejection of birth control – at least before the First World War - was its origins in prostitution.[31] This is difficult to appreciate, now that condoms are placed next to the check out in chemists and petrol stations, on supermarket shelves next to children's medicines, or in women's public toilets (even chocolate flavoured condoms in family toilet facilities); where children can watch 'hard core' pornography on videos, or 'soft core' pornography on the TV. It is hard to imagine a society where it was thought necessary to protect children from the knowledge of adult sexual practices, let alone from the ideology that children are a financial burden from which adults should be protected. An advertisement of 1796 makes plain the origins of artificial birth control, for any with lingering doubts:

"This advertisement is to inform our customers and others, that the woman who pretended the name of Philips, in Orange-court, is now dead, and that the business is carried on at Mrs. PHILIPS's WAREHOUSE, That has been for forty years, at the Green Canister, in Bedford (late Half-Moon) Street, seven doors from the Strand, on the left hand side, STILL continues in its original state of reputation; where all gentlemen of intrigue may be supplied with those Bladder Policies, or implements of safety, which infallibly secure the health of our customers…N.B. Ambassadors, foreigners, gentlemen and captains of ships, &c. going abroad, may be supplied with any quantity of the best goods in England, on the shortest notice…"[32]

There is no lack of clues to the true origins of birth control; indeed, we must thank birth control historians for setting them out so plainly. However, later feminist interpretations have glossed over the misogynist roots of the birth control campaign to such an extent that it is now perceived as a feminist campaign for women's freedom from children. This process has been aided by our own, erroneous, perceptions of those whose lifestyle and philosophy were totally different,[33] meaning that even the most glaring evidence can be overlooked. It is relatively easy for the casual enquirer to swallow the line that historical evidence of contraceptive use points to a desire on the part of the mass of ancient women to avoid pregnancy, when it is far more likely to be evidence of methods used by prostitutes and temple priestesses to prevent pregnancy and thus avoid interruption to their occupation.

In truth, up to relatively recently, contraceptives have been used because of *men's* desire to avoid pregnancy, for which they would be financially responsible. Thus, the Banks, in *Feminism and Family Planning in Victorian England,* while noting the higher age of marriage as a factor in falling birth rates, fail to draw similar conclusions from the falling infant mortality rate. Likewise Peter Fryer, in *The Birth Controllers,* while dwelling on a bizarre range of birth control methods, fails to mention the infant mortality rate. In one way, at least, Bradlaugh and Besant were successful. They encouraged the development of a society in which the advent of children was no longer seen as part of normal life, but looked upon simply as an unfortunate by-product of sex.

Killing- Always With Us?

Historians of birth control dwell on routine infanticide,[34] to show that population control has always been with us and that if the birth control professionals were not on hand, people would use other, more brutal methods of controlling their fertility.[35] They suggest that such practices have always been carried out to limit the numbers of children for reasons of economy, with abortion and infanticide part of a 'natural tendency', carried out because primitive peoples had no access to contraception.

The attitude of birth control historians towards the killing of babies has been one of cold, scientific detachment, verging on the voyeuristic. For example, having spent a great deal of time assuring his bemused reader that ancient peoples had always practised infanticide to keep down their numbers, Norman Himes confidently asserts: "There can be no doubt but that infanticide has contributed to group survival in a certain state of cultural evolution. This is not to say that we need it now. We do not, for we have a reliable substitute."[36]

Any reliable historical evidence of the practice of homicide may show that these events were the exception rather than the rule. Undoubtedly, these things happened – but not necessarily for the reasons alleged by birth control historians. In the absence of firm information, however, we are led to assume that it was pre-historic 'couples' deciding on such a course of action, and carrying it out – but were they really the culprits? The historians are coy about exploring exactly *who* was responsible for infanticide in ancient times. But as Linda Gordon admits: "These are women's choices, but hardly choices coming from positions of power.[37]

It is unlikely that the less powerful sex in an ancient community would kill their own children in opposition to the wishes of powerful leaders, simply to exercise 'choice'. If they did, it must have been at the behest of men. If they killed their babies for reasons of economy – as alleged - would they have done so willingly, or under duress?[38]

Since children would have been responsible for the welfare of their parents in old age (the traditional fear of which has always haunted the poor), it seems unlikely that killing babies would really have been seen as an economy. A large number of children would surely have been seen as an old age insurance policy. The fact that few survived would be more likely the result of harsh living conditions, than a deliberate attempt to sustain some sort of idyllic prehistoric lifestyle, as Stopes imagined with her flower-wreathed love-making. It is highly unlikely that early women, in an attempt to 'control their fertility', resorted habitually to infanticide - though that is not to say that infanticide did not occur for other reasons than modern feminist rhetoric would suggest.

Germaine Greer, in *Sex and Destiny*, appears to show ambivalence to these ancient methods of 'fertility control', alleging that the Yanomamo Indians practised infanticide *and* abortion, but that many women underwent abortion rather than commit infanticide, "which was not, and probably never has been, taken lightly." [39]

However, the assertion that women never took infanticide lightly is difficult to square with her description of such methods 'traditionally' employed: "She herself may have bashed its brains out with a rock, or thrown it on the ground or against a tree, or strangled it with a vine or stood upon a stick laid across its neck or poured sand into its mouth. Such violent acts were the more merciful…"[40] Greer implies that such violence indicates a darker side to motherhood, and claims: "…the great affection of infanticidal peoples for their surviving children is quite understandable."[41]

Communities that habitually murdered their children may well have been happy, well-adjusted groups; however, the impression is given that *women* commit such crimes, not because their minds, or their hormones, are unbalanced, but because their books will not balance. Their motives are purely mercenary, it is alleged, and they can put aside the murder of a newborn infant without so much as a tear. (Leaving aside the possibility of another pregnancy ensuing, because lactation has ceased.)

If such poor people thought only in cold, rational, selfish terms, it is important to remember that children represented security in old age. Any study of a society which values males above females (such as China, where sons are responsible for their parents' upkeep in old age, and bride-trafficking has become a serious problem because of a shortage of females),[42] will prefer boys. But girls are still necessary to help in the home, even if we ignore the fact that poor people value their children for reasons other than purely mercenary ones.

In ancient societies, especially agrarian ones, people actually worshipped fertility. In today's society, where women are encouraged to see their fertility as something to be restrained, it is hard to imagine a society where fertility was actually welcomed. In certain circumstances, e.g. war, famine, etc., cannibalism of children has occurred, though it has hardly been looked upon as a goal of feminism or a social blessing.

Human *sacrifice* of some sort has also been a feature of human societies from early times, though more widely among agricultural communities than pastoral or hunting peoples (the latter so beloved of birth control historians, because they were said to abandon any weaklings who could not keep up). It was believed that the blood of the sacrifice made the soil more fertile. Paradoxically, the human being - the most highly valued - was considered the best material for sacrifice.[43] But serious historians do not imply that women whose babies were torn from their arms for sacrificial purposes, gave up their children willingly in the name of female empowerment, or 'choice'.

Only in 1836 did it become law for British deaths to be officially registered, following widespread alarm over cases of secret poisoning. The absence of outward signs of violence on a corpse, it was said, might nevertheless conceal murder. A number of books on forensic medicine became available in the English language in the 1830s warning of these dangers, and in 1836 an Act was passed which authorised coroners for the first time to pay for post-mortem examinations. The registering of deaths provided a useful check on those not accounted for in burial registers – over 44,000 - and made it harder to conceal a death.

A great scandal in early Victorian times was the practice of enrolling children in 'burial clubs' that paid out a sum of money on their death. Chadwick asserted that these clubs provided "a bounty on neglect and infanticide."[44] Here there would appear to be a positive incentive for the unscrupulous to kill their children. However, it would be difficult to prove that such parents murdered their children because they had no access to contraception.

Another grim by-product of the workhouse system was the practice of unmarried mothers boarding their infants with 'baby-farmers'. Such mothers would have to decide whether to stay in the workhouse, earning their living by cleaning and other hard work - in which case they would be separated from the child – or leaving the workhouse with a two-week-old baby, and taking their chances. The Poor Law Guardians were supposed to protect the babies by visiting the homes where they were boarded by their mothers while they took employment but despite this, much indirect infanticide took place, as Emmeline Pankhurst relates:

"...under the law, if a man who ruins a girl pays down a lump sum of twenty pounds...the boarding home is immune from inspection. As long as a baby-farmer takes only one child at a time, the twenty pounds being paid, the inspectors cannot inspect the house. Of course the babies die with hideous promptness, often long before the twenty pounds have been spent, and then the baby-farmers are free to solicit another victim."[45]

Feminists rejected Malthusian claims that birth control would do away with such tragedies. They preferred economic and political remedies instead. However, even when these appalling scandals were stamped out, birth control advocates still made capital out of infanticide. So many children died in infancy anyway that it was an easy claim to make, and one that was difficult to check or disprove.

In fact, it was not until 1915 that parents and medical attendants were legally obliged to notify all births. It is still possible to surmise that before this time, because of the lack of contraception, many babies were murdered in secret. But there were also thousands of abandoned infants, as well as unmarried mothers who gave birth in the Workhouse because they had nowhere else to go. Murder was not, even in the harshest of circumstances, inevitable. We must therefore presume that the tendency to murder was, and remains, confined to a small minority of the population whose minds or morals are disordered.

If infanticide was evenly spread throughout the community, the human race would hardly have survived – especially in times of hardship when, the Malthusians alleged, parents resorted to infanticide for reasons of subsistence. It is in times of hardship that the parental bond that dictates extreme self-sacrifice in order to promote a child's welfare, tightens rather than loosens.

Widespread secret infanticide could be only be alleged by the Malthusians when many babies were dying in infancy anyway. If there were only a handful of such cases, they would have had to justify their claim.[46] However, when the infant mortality rate began to come down in the better-off classes, William Beveridge (later architect of the Welfare state), still claimed that the "revolutionary fall in fertility during the last fifty years was due in the main to practices as deliberate as infanticide."[47] It is interesting that, a decade or so later, similar allegations were to be made about poor women concealing large numbers of abortions.

The indifference of birth control pioneers to the suffering and death of innocent babies, and their use of tragic cases to promote birth control, gives a further clue to their main aim. It was not to ease suffering, but to control population.

Birth control historians' preoccupation with warnings about abortion gives the modern reader an unintended insight into people's traditional abhorrence of birth control *and* abortion, and also illustrates the attitudes of the historians themselves. In their sympathetic handling of the birth control pioneers' indifference to such tragedies as abortion and infanticide, they illustrate their own preoccupation with population control. Many such historians were, in fact, part of the birth control movement.

Norman Himes, for example, was a member of the Population Association of America.[48] Dr Clive Wood, author of books on sex, fertility and birth control, was involved in studying intrauterine devices. Beryl Suitters worked for International Planned Parenthood (IPPF).[49] Audrey Leathard was Vice-Chair of North Exeter Family Planning Association.[50] Dr Peter Diggory has been involved in the Doctors and Overpopulation Group. Dr Malcolm Potts has been Medical Director of the IPPF. Elizabeth Draper was "secretary and investigator" to a research group set up to advise the Family Planning Association on "how its work might be 'brought further into line with present requirements'".[51]

Crucially, much historical material on the birth control movement has been supplied by its own pioneers: people such as Edith Summerskill, Dora Russell, Lena Jeger, Mary Stocks, Lela Sargent Florence, and, of course, Stopes and Sanger. Their involvement in, and sympathy with, the birth control movement, should be taken into account when evaluating their histories, as should the standpoint of any author. The danger is that more recent books, drawing on these earlier works, tend to reflect their views without the reader being aware of the standpoints of the original writers. The motivations of the birth controllers are subject to less scrutiny, and their less pleasant aspects ignored, or downplayed. This is how history can easily be distorted.

For example, one book on women's health claimed: "In 1882 the diaphragm was invented; an important year both for the history of contraception and for the liberation of women." However, the feminist authors fail to mention that the inventor was a Malthusian – indeed, there is no mention of Malthusianism at all.[52]

Another point to remember is that studies which focus on one narrow aspect of people's lives can result in a very narrow perspective on history. In this respect, studies like that of Elizabeth Roberts, on Lancashire women, is concerned with whole lives, and perhaps for this reason, rings true.

How Popular was Birth Control?

Birth control historians list many campaigning groups in the 1920s, which seem to show how much popular agitation there was for birth control. There was the National Birth Control Association (NBCA); the National Birth Control Council (NBCC); the New Generation League; the Society for Constructive Birth Control and Racial Progress (SCBC); the Society for the Provision of Birth Control Clinics (SPBCC); the Birth Control International Information Centre (BCIIC). There was even a Workers' Birth Control Group (WBCG).[53]

But many birth control campaigners were involved in more than one group. Lady Denman, for example, was Chair of the NBCC and also chaired the Executive Committee of the NBCA. She was a supporter of the SPBCC and later was involved in the Family Planning Association (FPA). Margaret Pyke was involved in the NBCC and NBCA; later she would be involved in the FPA and the International Planned Parenthood Federation (IPPF).[54]

The groups often collaborated, sharing aims and objectives, but each working its own 'territory'. A number of birth control campaigners were involved with, or helped to found, birth control clinics, as a practical way of furthering the cause. These voluntary clinics did not all reflect their preoccupation in their names.[55]

For example, Margery Spring-Rice (involved in the BCIC and NBCC) was also Chair of the Ladbroke Grove Clinic. Margaret Pyke helped to found the Plymouth Clinic. Mary Stocks co-founded the Manchester and Salford Mother's Clinic. Dr Helena Wright (involved in the NBCC and NBCA, and later the FPA and IPPF) worked for the North Kensington Clinic.[56] The clinics were an inseparable part of the birth control campaign. They were concrete expressions of the beliefs of the birth control priests and priestesses, a practical way of spreading their gospel, even when that gospel remained unpreached to the flock at whom it was aimed - the poor.

Those who were members of political parties or women's organisations took the battle for birth control into those organisations, helping to shape policy. Lady Denman and Margery Spring-Rice worked for birth control within the Liberal Party. Leah L'Estrange Malone, Ruth Dalton, Joan Allen and Margaret Lloyd, members of the WBCG, worked within the Labour Party and the Independent Labour Party. Eva Hubback, already involved in the NBCA and NBCC (and later with the FPA) worked tirelessly for birth control within the feminist umbrella organisation, the National Union of Societies for Equal Citizenship (NUSEC), alongside the WBCG and SPBCC. Stella Browne, a well-known feminist writer, agitated for birth control within the Communist Party. Mary Stocks, a friend of Hubback's, was involved in the National Council of Women (NCW) and NUSEC. Lela Sargent Florence was involved in the National Council for Equal Citizenship.[57] Margery Spring-Rice was involved in the Women's National Liberal Federation. Edith How-Martyn was honorary secretary of the Women's Social and Political Union (WSPU).[58]

After the Ministry of Health edict of 1930, a plethora of organisations was no longer needed. The National Birth Control Council was formed in the same year to co-ordinate the existing groups, and the energy that had characterised the birth control movement found expression in the movement for sterilisation. The WBCG and the Birth Control Investigation Committee (the latter was formed in 1927 to study birth control techniques and use) merged with the NBCC in 1930 and 1931 respectively. The SPBCC and the BCIIC both merged fully with the NBCA (as the NBCC became in 1931) in 1938. Efforts to assimilate Marie Stopes' campaign with the other organisations failed. In 1939, the organisations ceased to function separately. Reflecting the general fears of a dwindling birth rate in their new name, they became the Family Planning Association.[59]

Like a chameleon, the birth control campaign went through many confusing changes, but still remained essentially the same, its true Malthusian colours well concealed. The Society for the Provision of Birth Control Clinics (SPBCC), which helped organise the great public conference in 1930 calling for birth control information to be given by local authority clinics, and later merged with the NBCA was, in fact, the name adopted by the Walworth Women's Welfare Centre in 1924. How did this 'Welfare Centre' begin? In 1921, it started life as the birth control clinic of the Malthusian League, which, in an effort to project a more positive image, later changed its name to the New Generation League.[60]

The SPBCC (whose sympathisers included Lady Denman), raised money, and encouraged the formation of new clinics – at North Kensington, Wolverhampton, Cambridge, Manchester and Salford, East London, Glasgow, Aberdeen and Oxford.[61] Involved with the North Kensington Clinic were Margaret Lloyd (of the WBCG), Mrs Rollo Russell (Margaret Lloyd's mother, who helped with the loan of premises at Ladbroke Grove), and Margery Spring-Rice (Chair of the Clinic). Also involved were Margaret Pollock, a friend of Lloyd's, and Dr Joan Malleson. Both these were members of the Malthusian League (Pollock was a Vice-President). Malthusian influence even reached into government. Another WBCG member, Ruth Dalton, wife of MP Hugh Dalton, was on the executive committee of the SPBCC.[62]

The modern twentieth century birth control campaign which, we are led to assume, had 'shaken off' its dusty, Malthusian image, was directly influenced by Malthusians, its aims being influenced by Malthusian belief. But, like bank robbers fleeing the scene of the crime, a number of changes of vehicle ensured a clean getaway.

The Tragedy of Poor Women

Another active birth control campaigner whose story has been well told is Elizabeth Daniels. Daniels, a health visitor for Edmonton council, was dismissed in 1922 for giving out birth control information, after a warning by her Medical Officer. Her case became yet another birth control campaign *cause célèbre*, as the great and the good of the birth control movement[63] took it up and ran with it.

As Audrey Leathard puts it: "[Miss Daniels]…had been dismissed from her post, as health visitor with Edmonton District Council, for giving birth control advice. Despite previous warning, 'the tragedy of poor women she visited proved too much for her, and she determined to help them'."[64] But there was a little more to it than that. Nurse Daniels was a Malthusian, and the birth control 'information' she handed out consisted of the addresses of the Marie Stopes clinic and the New Generation League.

She became the focus for the political campaign for disseminating birth control information on the rates.[65] For as Soloway puts it: "They [the birth control campaigners] compared the meager accomplishments of their sixteen or seventeen clinics, most open only a few hours a week, with the enormous potential of the more than 2,200 local infant and maternal welfare clinics closed to them by ministerial decree".[66]

The hoped-for flood of poor women into the birth control clinics had turned out to be a disappointing trickle. No doubt it occurred to Daniels that she could accelerate the process. During the storm occasioned by her dismissal, she went to Holland to learn about Mensinga diaphragms, and returned to open a (private) clinic, where the Dutch methods were taught to nurses.[67]

What of her feelings for the "tragedy of poor women"? Soloway records that she found her work "frustrating". Apparently "...patients were frequently ignorant and unappreciative. Nurse Daniels complained that when women discovered that they had to buy and insert the Mensinga diaphragm themselves since they were not 'charms' that worked magically without any effort on their part, they often left."

Unconsciously revealing her true feelings towards "poor women", she claimed that results were more encouraging among those she termed "the wives of less 'primitive' workers". She said that many women came to the clinic at their husbands' urging. It was usually the men who initiated the correspondence.[68] A few years later, she was advertising for private custom in the *New Generation* as "late health visitor, Edmonton".[69]

From the beginning, the birth controllers wanted to limit the numbers of the poor. They claimed to have compassion for poor people, and some even came to believe their own rhetoric. But, as we have seen, the poor were suspicious - and rightly so - of the motives of these self-invited friends. The Malthusian claim that they were dedicated to the 'elimination of poverty' was seen by some as a dedication to eliminate the poor. But when confronted by antagonism, the Malthusians protested their political neutrality.[70]

It soon became obvious from attacks by 'rabid socialists' that a body representing the interests of the wealthy and the middle classes, would never succeed in influencing the poor. Though their influence may have been small, and downplayed by historians,[71] opponents such as the Marxist Social Democratic Federation had powerful arguments. They blamed the plight of the poor, not on the poor themselves, but on the rich. Their arguments fatally undermined the Malthusians' credibility with those they were trying to save.

As Soloway puts it: "The first Neo-Malthusians knew that they would have to overcome an entrenched legacy of working-class antipathy toward Malthus. He and his philosophical heirs had long been denounced as enemies of the poor because their laissez-faire ideas epitomized the self-serving rationalizations of the propertied classes. The likelihood of persuading working people that their difficulties were a consequence of their own thoughtless fertility rather than the entrenched inequities of economic and political institutions was further complicated by the rapid emergence in the 1880s of socialism and a more aggressive trade unionism".[72]

While the female birth controllers went to work on poor women, the males concentrated on poor men, in a way that confirmed the suspicion of working-class activists. The Honorary Secretary of the New Generation League, Dr Binnie Dunlop, writing in the *Daily Telegraph* in 1924, enthused:

"The wage-earners know that increased production alone will not bring them the standard of living which they rightly aspire to, and the only alternative they hear of is Socialism or Revolution. If, however, they were given the doctrine of increased production plus controlled reproduction, they would quickly be won over to the capitalist system".[73]

However, James Maxton, MP, writing in the left-wing *New Leader*, says:

"The birth controllers in the Labour and Socialist movement have never found me a protagonist of their theories. It always seemed to me quite irrelevant to the Socialist theory. It placed the responsibility for poverty on the numbers in the population rather than on the maldistribution of goods, and suggested that if there were fewer people there would be more wealth for each individual.

"I believe this to be profoundly untrue in a capitalist society, and akin to the view of the temperance enthusiasts that drink is the cause of poverty.

"My own philosophy of life makes me believe that an intelligent control of the appetites and desires, both in food and drink and sex, is productive of greater personal usefulness than the unbridled indulgence of these. But these personal predilections do not form a foundation for a Socialist policy, and the idea that in a capitalist state of society teetotalism or having no children would do anything to solve the poverty problem is a fantastic one."[74]

With these and similar arguments exposing the Malthusians' 'campaign against poverty', it was time for the birth controllers to figuratively throw aside the "grimy mantle of Malthus"[75] and struggle into working clothes, as Annie Besant had done literally in the nineteenth century. By entering the political fray, they could fight the 'rabid socialists' on their own ground, using arguments of equality and compassion to prove their point, as had Besant with *her* socialist friends. As it turned out, they were to have more success than she did.

Apart from a small number of 'co-operators' who had always been sympathetic to birth control,[76] the labour movement on the whole was antagonistic or indifferent. As Leathard admits: "Labour members disliked Drysdale's Malthusian 'adherence to the more dismal aspects of economics' and were emotionally repelled by the idea of contraception."[77] She goes on

69

(somewhat ironically, given the male-supremacy stance of Malthusianism): "Birth control activists were totally middle-class; the bulk of the Labour Party support came from the male-orientated working class."[78]

The best way to influence labour organisations was to actually work from within, and this is what the birth control advocates did. Stella Browne, Janet Chance, Edith How-Martyn, Eva Hubback, Frida Laski, Leah L'Estrange Malone, Joan Malleson, Dora Russell, Dorothy Thurtle, Cicely Hamilton, Dorothy Jewson, Rose Witcop, Margaret Lloyd, Alice Hicks and Joan Allen, all with birth control affiliations, worked within the socialist political parties. Most were members of the WBCG.

Some were personal friends. Laski, L'Estrange Malone, Malleson, and Allen, were all friends of Dora Russell.[79] (Margaret Pollock was a friend of Margaret Lloyd, cousin of Dora's husband Bertrand Russell.) Dorothy Jewson, President of the WBCG, was returned as MP for Norwich. Jenny Adamson was the wife of Labour MP, W. M. Adamson. Dorothy Thurtle, on the Committee of the WBCG, was the daughter of George Lansbury, and wife of Ernest Thurtle, Labour MP for Shoreditch in the East End of London. Joan Allen was married to Clifford Allen (later Baron Hurtwood), a Labour MP who went on to found the all-Party 'Next Five Years Group'.[80]

Ruth Dalton – a member of the Malthusian SPBCC, as we have noted - was the wife of Dr Hugh Dalton, Labour President of the Board of Trade. According to Audrey Leathard, Ruth Dalton used her influence within the Independent Labour Party to further the cause of birth control, as an executive member of the WBCG. During the Second World War, when raw materials vital to the war effort were in short supply, birth control advocates were alarmed that not enough rubber was being made available for contraceptive manufacture. Leathard relates "…Lord Horder" [first President of the NBCA] was in touch with the President of the Board of Trade, Dr Dalton,[81] whose wife Ruth was an active family planner. By the end of 1944 the authorities relented; enough rubber could be released to supply doctors, including those at clinics, with appliances for their patients".[82]

Such friendships must have made it easier to discuss the strategy of the birth control campaign within the Labour Party. Dora Russell, recalling dinner parties held in her Chelsea home during the Twenties, says: "…among political friends, the L'Estrange Malones, Hugh and Ruth Dalton, Harold and Frida Laski were not far away and frequent visitors".[83]

Strange Bed-Fellows

Birth control historians have been able to point to left-wing birth control activists to prove that birth control has been historically in the interests of women and the poor.

However, when it is revealed that these radicals were at the same time working with the archconservatives of the population control movement, ready excuses have been found for them. Of Edith How-Martyn and her husband, Soloway says: "They were rare catches indeed for that organization. [the

Malthusian League] But when they joined in 1910 it was not out of any sympathy with the league's individualistic economic philosophy, which, as members of the Independent Labour party, they frankly deplored. The How-Martyns, like several other social reformers, grudgingly allied with the league before the war simply because there was no other organization promoting family limitation, and it was clear that neither the suffrage groups nor the fledgling Labour party were about to take it up."[84] In *Politics of Motherhood*, Jane Lewis says: "Two feminists, Eva Hubback and Edith How-Martyn did join the [Malthusian] league in 1910, but were never very active because they disliked the classical economic doctrines it espoused".[85]

Why, if people like Hubback and the How-Martyns were so convinced of the vital importance of birth control to social reform, did they not set up their own organisation? After all, feminist Sylvia Pankhurst had done the same when, as a pacifist - and unlike other Suffragettes - she had disagreed with the First World War. Clearly, there must have been greater advantages in working within existing political organisations. And, though Soloway claims that some birth control advocates "allied with the organization because, until 1921, there was no other dedicated to the promotion of smaller families among the distressed poor",[86] the truth is, many were still members of these reactionary organisations after 1921 - in fact, they supported several organisations, as we have seen.

Soloway says of Stella Browne: "[she] decided to use the offices of the [Malthusian] league, confident she could get her message across to labouring women without it being polluted by the laissez-faire, utilitarian nonsense usually spouted by the organization's orthodox propagandists".[87]

This – if it were true - must have been merely wishful thinking. The views expressed by the Malthusians, both within and without their magazine, make it difficult to see how self-proclaimed defenders of justice for the poor could work with, or support, the Malthusians, who had frequently made it clear whose side *they* were on in the class war. And of course, the "labouring women" for whose welfare Browne was so solicitous, were not likely to read a copy of the *Malthusian*.

Admittedly, the *Malthusian* applauded the lengthy dock strike of 1889 – but only because it drew attention to the problem of surplus labour![88] In other words, there were 'too many' poor people, jostling for a limited number of jobs. Strikes, they believed, were the inevitable result.

Their attitude to immigration was even less compassionate. Most of the Neo-Malthusians were "strongly opposed to the influx of aliens, many of them Eastern European Jews, in the late nineteenth and early twentieth centuries…Occasionally Malthusian League members succumbed to nativist passions and fulminated against the 'filthy scum and refuse' dumped on Britain's shores, and they sometimes endorsed the use of force to eject these 'starving barbarians' who represented 'not the survival of the fittest, but the unfittest.'"[89]

The Malthusian League believed that these immigrants were victims not of oppression, but of over-population. In a move which finds echoes in modern

China, C. R. Drysdale and his wife Alice Vickery Drysdale tried to persuade their colleagues to sponsor a 'Malthusian statute' based on John Stuart Mill's maxim, that the state should "guarantee ample employment to all who are born" in return for assurances that "no person shall be born without its consent". The Drysdales were prepared to enforce this statute with fines and a denial of poor relief if couples exceeded their allotted number of children.[90] According to Soloway the League, at C V Drysdale's urging, "not only condemned school meals and medical examinations for the poor, but old age pensions, improved workmen's compensation, better housing, and national health insurance..." The League also condemned universal adult suffrage.[91]

According to the *Malthusian*, C V Drysdale was anti-immigration, and opposed to militant labour. He wanted strikes to be made illegal.[92] In 1915, after a series of wage demands, strikes and slowdowns, C V Drysdale attacked the "traitorous, socialist-run trade unions and the 'cowardly and weak' politicians who posed a greater threat to the nation than the Kaiser."[93] Incredibly, despite Drysdale's anti-Left fulminations, the socialist Stella Browne "drew on his work".[94]

Bessie Drysdale, C V's wife, "shared his abiding hatred of collectivism and socialism".[95] While writing heart-wrenching stories about poor unwanted "bybies" in the *New Generation* magazine, she believed in *compulsory* birth control for the poor: "Another byby? Well, I think I'll clear out. There ain't a bit of peace and quiet in this 'ouse wot with one kid or another always yellin'. Wot we want 'ere is more vittles an' less kids."[96]

While the Malthusians were frequently guilty of blurting out their true feelings, their 'socialist' and 'feminist' allies were more cautious. As Soloway puts it: "Class arguments, though often confused with feminist goals, were always more central to the Workers Birth Control Group."[97] In other words, they used the rhetoric of socialism and feminism to achieve exactly the same goal: fewer poor people. The 'socialists' appealed to class envy, declaring that birth control should be available to the working classes, not just the middle classes, while 'feminists' declared that women should have the freedom to choose motherhood. They employed Besant's tactic of using 'compassionate' arguments when debating with socialists.

Unlike Christians, socialists and social reformers of all political parties, the Malthusians did not believe in ameliorating the conditions of the poor, since they believed that the cause of poverty was overpopulation. Any form of charity would simply exacerbate the situation,[98] because it would encourage the poor to breed. C V Drysdale, himself a doctor, in his testimony to the National Birth Rate Commission,[99] refused to concede that the efforts of physicians over the previous forty years had had any effect whatsoever on mortality.

He stubbornly clung to the belief that it was the decline of the *birthrate* (accomplished, as he saw it, in the teeth of medical opposition), which had resulted in a lower death rate: "No new medical skills nor hygienic advances could account for so dramatic a fall".[100] According to Soloway: "He told the incredulous commissioners that the fall in fertility was solely responsible for the improvement [in infant mortality]. Recent strides in public health and the control of childhood disease had no effect whatsoever.... 'So rigidly do I conclude it, that I do not believe sanitation or medicine or any of these great advances have as yet...saved a life at all.'".[101]

It is difficult to believe that any true socialist or feminist could tolerate working with the holders of such reactionary views, but on closer examination, the 'radical' proponents of birth control do not come up smelling of roses, either. We find even Annie Besant larding her exhortations to use birth control, with threats:

"The first upward step towards that happier life will only be taken when parents resolutely determine to limit their family to their means, and *stamp with disapproval every married couple who selfishly overcrowd their home, to the injury of the community of which they are a part*.

(My italics)[102]

The battle in the Labour Party over permitting local authorities to give contraceptive advice at their maternity clinics, has been well told in birth control histories. The main actor in the drama was Dora Russell, whom we have already encountered. Russell (also a member of the Independent Labour Party and the Malthusian League) has related the story of her 'battle for birth control' at length, in her autobiography, 'The Tamarisk Tree'. [103]

A deputation of birth control advocates presented a petition of six thousand signatures to the Labour Minister of Health in 1924, calling for birth control advice to be available to mothers.[104] It proved unsuccessful. Motions were put to the annual Labour Party Conference by local party branches. Attempts were made to vote on the issue, and so make it part of official party policy. The battle rumbled on but, when the Labour Government fell in 1924, the Ministerial ban on birth control advice from public clinics – issued after the birth control deputation made its plea – was still intact.[105] This ban was to be kept firmly in place by the succeeding Conservative Government.

January 1924 – a few months before the birth control deputation - saw the election of the first-ever Labour government in Britain. Many poor people, still reeling from the effects of the First World War, were disillusioned by the capitalist system with its failed promises of 'homes fit for heroes'. With the end of the post-War boom, the industrial co-operation that had prevailed during the War was conveniently forgotten, and those who had helped Lloyd George to power saw an opportunity to cut wages and break the strength of the trade unions.

The mines were not, after all, to be nationalised, and the mine owners refused to negotiate wages on a national basis, insisting on piece-meal agreements. The miners would not accept this, wanting the better-off mines to subsidise the less well off. On March 31, the mine owners locked them out. The solidarity of the 'Triple Alliance' failed.[106] As the post-War slump began to bite, unemployment reached two millions. Trade union membership fell as members were thrown out of work. Trade union funds were depleted by unemployment benefit payments of over seven million pounds.

The birth control campaigners also had high hopes of the 1924 Election. The birth control issue had been successfully raised in the Women's Cooperative Guild Congress of 1923, and had narrowly missed similar discussion at the Labour Women's Conference of that year. In the following May, Dora Russell was a prominent member of the deputation presenting the petition to the new Minister of Health. Great play has been made of the anti-birth control stance of the Minister, John Wheatley, and his religion:

"...the Minister of Health...Mr Wheatley, who, unfortunately, was a Roman Catholic". (Russell)[107] "Marie Stopes warned that the new Minister of Health...was a Catholic." (Leathard)[108] "But Wheatley was a Roman Catholic." (Fryer)[109] "Unfortunately, the Minister of Health...was a Roman Catholic." (Lewis)[110] "The Minister, John Wheatley, a Catholic, was unsympathetic..." (Barbara Brookes)[111]

But there was more to the matter than religion. There was the fragile majority of the new, inexperienced Labour government to consider, and a fear of a split in the ranks. There was the large Catholic contingency in the Labour Party, and its supporters. And, what was obvious to people at the time - if not today - they needed more, not less, working-class voters. Solidarity, strength in numbers, cooperation; historically, these formed the bedrock of the labour movement. There was a real fear that all birth control could accomplish, would be to help the labouring classes to shrink. The Malthusians, with their right-wing rhetoric, had made the poor suspicious of birth control.

They were right to be suspicious. Marie Stopes, pondering on the problem of how to introduce the poor to birth control "...favored political neutrality and the persuasion of key individuals in each party".[112] But it was realised by the more astute, that the left-wing parties must be won over, because the poor tended to trust them. However, Malthusian rhetoric would not only antagonise left-wing politicians, but be construed by them as meaning fewer working-class votes. The poor would never be persuaded to use birth control if their political representatives were against it. It seemed an impossible situation. But Malthusian sympathisers in the labour and cooperative movements were not about to give up.

The Trojan Horse

The deputation to the Minister of Health was composed of representatives of the SCBC (Marie Stopes' organisation), and the New Generation League (formerly the Malthusian League), acting in a "rare display of cooperation".[113] H. Jennie Baker moved Dora Russell's pro-birth control addendum at the 1924 Labour Party Conference. Both were Malthusians. (Soloway says that Baker found it "impossible" to pass on the New Generation's paper, or to be "publicly associated" with the organisation, because of the Drysdales' remarks.)[114] The plain speaking of the old-fashioned Malthusians did not go down too well in the Labour movement, and at the Conference, Baker instead cited "tragic cases", asking, "whether mothers had not the right to prevent more misery being brought into the world".[115] Despite acknowledging the repellant nature of Malthusian rhetoric, Baker remained part of Marie Stopes' Society for Constructive Birth Control and Racial Progress.[116]

Many such arguments, even when they started with compassion, soon slid into Malthusianism and eugenics - even at Labour Party Conferences. The birth control debate at the 1927 conference heard the writer H. N. Brailsford, after giving heartrending individual stories illustrating the need for birth control, conclude: "The doctor might know almost to a certainty that the child she will bear, even if it survives, will be unhealthy. The case might be worse − the case might be that she or her husband was afflicted with some hereditary disease."[117]

A Mr S. J. Davies, of Willesden Borough Labour Party, claimed that, though there were a "number of people in the country who knew how and when not to reproduce" it was also true that "there were a vast number of people who did not know. They were told that their whole material existence was bound up in economic circumstances, and as he viewed economic circumstances he would draw their attention to a picture of a cuttlefish. Issuing from the body of that cuttlefish were a number of tentacles....and one of those was the burden of overpopulation."[118]

While Davies claimed that everyone had a right to birth control information, Dr Stella Churchill, of Brentford and Chiswick, while opposing the birth control motion because she did not think that the Maternal and Child Welfare Centres were the right places to give such advice, stated that she was in favour of giving the advice to all women who wanted it, but also "to some of those who did not want it..."[119] She was not alone in favouring compulsion.

Malthusian influence permeated every aspect of the birth control campaign within the Labour Party. F. A. Broad, the Labour MP for Edmonton, who introduced the birth control question into Parliament for the first time, was Vice-president of the Malthusian League.[120] The first Women's Section of a local Labour Party branch to urge a change in public policy on birth control, was Chelsea − Dora Russell's and Stella Browne's branch.[121] Indeed, Russell was in charge of the resolutions.[122] Both Russell and Browne were Malthusians. As Russell recalls: "We did not differ from Marie Stopes in the important central aim, namely to make birth control 'respectable' and remove it from the aura of rubber-goods shops and sniggering."[123]

Russell was a dramatic personality, who had toyed with the idea of going on the stage. In fact, recalling the political upheavals of 1924, she says: "For me personally 1924 had been a great year. There had been enough drama and platform performances to satisfy my theatrical instincts."[124] She certainly enjoyed playing to the gallery. Her wit and charm made her an invaluable asset to the birth control movement, and Stella Browne was able to state in the

Malthusian paper, *The New Generation*, that the Russells "...have already done more than any other persons to link up our cause with the Labour movement."[125] "Our cause" was, of course, the population control movement.

Newly elected Labour MP Dorothy Jewson - President of the WBCG - actually wrote reports on the Labour Party Conference birth control debates for *The New Generation*.[126] Another WBCG member, Cicely Hamilton, contributed frequently to *The New Generation*, and was still Vice-President of the Malthusian League in 1937.[127] Stella Browne was a regular columnist.[128]

Having noted the Malthusian links of members of the Workers' Birth Control Group, it is now possible to gain some insight into the reasons for its formation. It was established in the wake of the 1924 Labour Party Conference to sustain "the momentum built up within the Women's Sections of the Labour party to force the minister of health to soften his stand on the welfare clinics."[129] The name was deliberately chosen to distance the organisation from the Malthusians: "We now formed our Workers' Birth Control Group to make clear that we were working in and with the Labour Party and did not share the views of the extreme Malthusians..."[130] So states Russell. Predictably, the WBCG was immediately welcomed by the other birth control organisations. Soloway comments: "Several of them [members of the WBCG] were also in the CBC, or New Generation League, and the three organizations agreed to assail the government together whenever possible".[131]

The WBCG employed tactics of harassment in order to further their agenda. As Leathard says: "...Labour women appealed to all Labour and Independent Labour Party members to pressurise the Minister of Health into action".[132] "[D]eputations descended on Wheatley".[133] Soloway relates: "Witcop, Russell, Stella Browne, Laski, Cicely Hamilton, and others kept up a steady assault on the leadership."[134]

Russell relates: "Meantime Dorothy Jewson and Ernest Thurtle were harassing him [John Wheatley] with questions in the House." Amused, she recalls: "Mr Wheatley had stirred a hornet's nest: all through 1924 we buzzed and stung."[135] They targeted Labour MPs who had voted against a Parliamentary Bill on birth control: "We got out a leaflet giving the names of Labour MPs who had voted for or against Mr Thurtle's Bill, [concerning local authority provision of contraception] and urged our supporters to tackle them".[136]

Any opposition was rejected, often with accusations of sexism.[137] But other objections were harder to brush away. Unwittingly betraying her own elitism (and, given her self-proclaimed feminism, her readiness to exploit the traditional bastions of male power), Russell reveals how she "sounded out" Members of Parliament, doctors and medical officers who were favourable to birth control, and "public men who might bring pressure to bear":

"The Independent Labour Party was especially inclined towards us: hence I once invited the Clydeside MPs, Campbell Stephen and Jimmy Maxton, to come to tea and discuss the matter. To my amusement they refused, implying that they did not wish to be accused of hobnobbing with the aristocracy.'"[138] When they did eventually meet, she was accused of "wanting to throw the baby out with the bath water: they were, naturally, resentful of the attitude of the Eugenists, who implied that the working classes should not breed because they were of inferior stock."

Unconsciously betraying her own attitudes, she continues: "It was perfectly true that, owing to women's ignorance, the workers had the largest families."[139] Maxton's later thoughts on the issue of birth control have already been noted, and it was John Wheatley who led the left-wing Clydeside group of MPs. Evidently the Scots were a much more suspicious body: when Margaret Sanger met with socialist men in Glasgow, in 1920, she found them "ready to fight the ancient battle of Marx against Malthus".[140]

Barbara Brookes records working-class reactions to Bertrand and Dora Russell's birth control campaign: "…they encountered opposition from workers who connected birth control with eugenics, and argued that what workers needed was more money and not fewer children".[141] Dora's flippant reply, that "…even if we lived in Buckingham Palace, we would not want a baby every year"[142] would hardly have soothed the irritation of her critics, especially when she was married to an Earl.

The Reverend James Barr, Labour MP for Motherwell, who debated with Dora on the birth control issue, accused Dora and Bertie of being "middle-class infiltrators into the Labour movement".[143]

As frustrating as the antagonism of the Left, must have been the support the birth control activists received from the Right. When Rose Witcop opened her 'People's Clinic' in London, "[m]uch to her astonishment she even received encouragement from the local Conservative paper".[144] Happy as they were to work privately with the reactionary forces in the birth control movement, it must have been embarrassing to have their right-wing support so blatantly advertised.

A similar embarrassment awaited Ernest Thurtle, Labour MP and husband of Dorothy (both supporters of the WBCG), when in 1926 he introduced a Bill permitting local authorities to provide free birth control instruction at their public welfare centres. The Bill was defeated by 167 votes to 82, with forty-six Labour MPs voting against. As Soloway remarks: "To add to the indignity, twice as many Conservatives as Labour members went into the division lobby with Thurtle."[145]

The Bandwagon Slows

With such a fragile majority in the Commons, and with so much work to do to improve the lives of the poor, it was understandable that the new Labour Government should have been wary of alienating any section of the electorate by embracing such a contentious issue as birth control. Many commentators have missed the point that if poor people did limit their families, not only would it not improve their incomes, but also it would result in a shrinking working class with even less industrial 'clout'. This prospect could hardly be expected to appeal to a Party struggling for its political life.

Large votes at the Party Conference in 1926 resulted in a victory for birth control. However, the position – resulting from the millions of votes cast by Trade Unions on behalf of members – was reversed in 1928 (it is alleged) by Catholic behind-the-scenes intrigue, in capturing the Trade Union vote. According to Soloway: "James Sexton, Labour MP and member of the powerful Transport and General Workers' Union, doubted whether the National Labour Women's Conference and those who supported its resolutions knew much about working-class women in the real world". He was not the only speaker who accused birth control advocates of living in a "fool's paradise". He "bluntly warned that the Catholic men and women who returned a great many Labour members to parliament would never agree to the party sanctioning birth control in any form".[146]

It was Sexton's 27th Labour Party Conference, he stated. He had spent ten years urging the TUC of the necessity of a vigorous political Labour Party. He had watched it grow from a mere infant to a strong able-bodied man, and therefore was jealous, he said, about the introduction of any subject that would prevent its further growth.[147]

Labour women Katharine Glasier, who had fought for maternity leave, and Ethel Bentham, a champion of baby clinics before the First World War, also refused to support the birth control campaign;[148] Mrs Harrison Bell[149] and Dr Esther Rickards protested at the Party Conference of 1926, that birth control was a "side-issue".[150] Discussion of birth control was ruled out of order for three years. Despite claims of popular support within the Party, it is significant that when the birth control activists switched courses, the popular feeling subsided.

Soloway remarks: "As the opposition became better organized and the political explosiveness of the issue became apparent, support began to wane".[151] A change in feeling could also have come about by appeals from Labour Party leaders not to allow the birth control issue to split the Party. The Party, realising that it was fighting for its political life, did respond – but not those members who were leading birth control advocates. The Editor of *Labour Woman*, Dr Marion Phillips, pointed out that the birth control issue was divisive; that there was much disagreement among doctors and scientists on the subject. In time, such a programme might be justified, but "the central task of the Labour party was to win elections and pass legislation that would redistribute wealth in such a way as to eliminate problems attributed to overpopulation".[152]

Phillips was saying what the Labour party leadership wanted, of course; but she herself did not see birth control as a magic wand to be waved at the problems of the poor, or that it was an important central issue of socialism. In fact, in *Labour Woman*, she criticised Sanger and Stopes. This dismayed Dora Russell, who duly reported to Stopes that she saw Phillips as a "problem".[153]

As a member of Labour's executive committee, Phillips was anxious about the negative impact of the birth control issue on Labour's tiny majority. But the birth controllers continued their campaign. Undaunted by the fall of the first Labour government after only a few months, the General Strike, and growing poverty in the communities of the poor, they grew even more strident. Labour leader Ramsay MacDonald was forced to step in.

During the 1926 Labour party Conference, after desperate attempts to sideline the issue,[154] MacDonald told the Conference of his own worries about limiting families, his fears of Malthusian influence and the offensive economic policies of the Malthusian League. Ultimately, he appealed on political grounds. The birth control issue was divisive. It would expose the Party to disruption. He pleaded with birth control advocates to treat the issue as a personal one, and to stop "digging ditches" between women and the party.[155]

But the birth control advocates were undeterred, and the following year, the conciliatory Party loyalist, Arthur Henderson, pleaded for moderation. He pointed out that the Party was already weakened by the collapse of the General Strike, and that its chances in the next election would be damaged. But his "pleas for loyalty and unity were ignored".[156]

MacDonald, it is well known, joined in a National Government with political opponents, after a crisis during the next Labour government, elected in 1929. The crisis was precipitated by the Labour Ministers' reluctance to impose a cut in Unemployment Benefit. The coalition government imposed spending cuts, and economic turmoil followed. Parliament was dissolved, and in the Election that followed, the jubilant Tories won 471 seats. The Labour Party was reduced from 289 MPs, to forty-six.

MacDonald has ever since been regarded as a traitor within the Labour Party. It seemed that he cared more about the prestige of office than the Party, which, used to being attacked on all sides, considered loyalty to be paramount. However, Francis Williams, in his history of the early Labour Party, acknowledges that MacDonald was originally anxious to build a strong Party, working hard to win over the more timid trade unionists: "He had devoted himself to building what he was far-seeing enough to know was the type of organization most likely to give a Labour Party numerical and financial strength and a firm foundation of mass support".[157] It would seem that his opposition to birth control was originally influenced by his desire for a strong Labour Party.

The new Labour Party was only too aware of the numerical aspects of their power base to embrace birth control as a central tenet of socialism – though Mary Stocks, writing on 'Population' in the 1920s *Encyclopaedia of the Labour Movement*, succeeds in manipulating the aspirations of the Party into a threat, at the same time unconsciously revealing the Malthusians' fear of socialism: "…the more equitable distribution of wealth and the achievement of the tolerable universal life-standard at which the Labour Party aims are likely to add their quota of complication to the [population] problem….they will make greater demands on space. The great mass of workers will take up more room in the world; for they will demand, and, it is to be hoped, secure, their share of country holidays, motor-roads, tennis-courts, gardens, solitude and silence".[158]

In 1924, the poor were less likely to be dreaming of country holidays and tennis courts, than having enough to eat. In any event, the first Labour government (and its Catholic Minister of Health) had proved a disappointment to the birth control movement. It was hoped their Conservative successors would be more receptive to the idea of birth control since, according to Soloway, they "were not beholden to large numbers of Catholics for their majority". Even more optimistically, they reasoned that since Tory Ministers would have more than their Ministerial pay to rely on, unlike the Labour Ministers, they would not feel so inclined to do the "safe" rather than the "heroic" thing.[159]

Since the Thurtle Bill, birth controllers had been more sanguine about the House of Lords as an engine of change. However, they turned their attention to Wheatley's successor, Neville Chamberlain and, sidestepping democracy, demanded that he sign an order without going through the House of Commons. After Chamberlain declined, for political reasons, to sanction their demands for birth control advice 'on the rates', the New Generation League raised £900 for a campaign to persuade him to change his mind, distributing half a million leaflets - with the help of local Labour party branches, the Independent Labour Party, and the Women's Co-operative Guild.[160]

Realism was beginning to creep into the birth control campaign. Even Dora Russell acknowledged that her birth control victory at the Labour Conference in 1926 was a "hollow one", as "Labour was not in power..."[161] While still claiming to feel strongly that "[birth control advice] was an inalienable right of women on which Governments should take action, which they would never do so long as the work was done for them by charity", she nevertheless "gradually" withdrew from the political fight for birth control.[162] Herbert Morrison urged her to stand for election to the London County Council, but she decided to put her energies into sex reform and education.[163]

This was worlds away from the heady days of her 1926 Conference victory, when she had threatened to split the Party. The National Labour Women's Conference - which had been supportive of birth control - would consider forming a separate party, she warned, if the next Labour Minister of Health did not change the Ministry's directive on birth control.[164]

As Sheila Rowbotham says: "Birth controllers turned away from the socialist movement, gaining broader support from NUSEC and the Women's National Liberal Federation".[165] After a large public meeting organised by the birth control groups in 1930 (influenced by the Malthusian SPBCC), the Ministry of Health quietly issued a memorandum allowing birth control 'advice' to be given by public clinics – but on medical grounds. The campaigners quickly publicised the memorandum.

However, their battle was not quite won, for this permission - to dispense birth control advice, on request, to married women, for medical reasons - was not enough. Despite their original claim that they were demanding birth control advice for health reasons, the campaigners' real motive was for the poor to limit their families. Supposing poor women did *not* request it?

The NBCA swiftly moved to demand advice on birth control on *economic*, as well as health, grounds, and the NCW, the NCEC, the Women's Co-operative Guild and the Women's Liberal Association quickly backed them.[166] Ignoring the many cultural and personal reasons why women – even poor women - might not request such advice, the NBCA also wanted health professionals to raise the issue of birth control with those whom they described as too diffident to ask for themselves.[167]

Despite further problems with doctors who did not wish to be pressurised into certain forms of action where individual patients' needs were concerned, and Catholic protest over local authorities affiliating to birth control campaign organisations,[168] British compromise was employed. Opposition to birth control became marginalised and weakened. By 1939, the NBCA had become the Family Planning Association, and was finally looking forward to enjoying respectability. Unfortunately for them, with the outbreak of the Second World War, people's thoughts turned to other, more urgent, matters.

When later recalling her struggle for birth control in the Labour Party, Russell claimed that the "modern threat of overpopulation had not yet dawned"[169] yet her own conversion to population control pre-dated her conversion to socialism. Her interest in population began, in fact, as a student at Cambridge University – long before any political interest or involvement.[170] Stella Browne was a member of the Communist Party who left after she failed to convert them on the question of abortion on demand.[171] Dorothy Thurtle entered local government in Shoreditch with the sole aim of establishing birth control clinics.[172] Frida Laski did the same in Fulham.[173] So did Edith Summerskill, in Wood Green.[174]

Maternal Mortality

Such moves might be seen as a natural extension of women's concern for other women, expressed in the desire to share knowledge. Arguments used were generally those of compassion, and Dame Janet Campbell's Ministry of Health report on maternal mortality in 1924 was certainly used by birth controllers to make their point.[175] But there were many others who realised that, with a complete lack of antenatal care, servants and labour-saving devices – not to mention good food and decent housing – birth control would not solve poor women's problems. Working-class women were not simply middle-class women with more children. They lived in a completely different world.

The Labour Party publication 'Protect the Nation's Mothers', published in 1936, referred to the dreadful toll of maternal deaths. During the past generation, there had been a continuous and substantial fall in infant mortality and general death rates, with longer life spans. However there had been no corresponding decline in maternal mortality, described in the booklet as "monstrous", and a "tragic state of affairs". It went on to claim that "half the deaths could be prevented".

To the birth controllers in the Labour Party, the solution to the maternal mortality problem was self-evident. If women did not give birth, they could not die in childbirth. At the 1927 Party Conference, miner's wife Mrs Lawther from Blaydon, made an impassioned plea for birth control knowledge based on the dangers of childbirth. Addressing the miners, she reminded them that the women had "stood foursquare with you in your dispute" and went on to tell them that it was "four times as dangerous for a woman to bear a child as it is for you to go down a mine. You are seeking legislation to make your occupation safe; will you still go on allowing your wives to suffer under this [birth control advice] ban?"[176]

The notion of it being more dangerous to bear a child than to go down a mine created a vivid impression, and it succeeded in silencing discontent at the Conference. Anyone opposing the campaign to overturn the Ministerial ban would henceforth be suspected of not caring about the dangers women faced from unwanted pregnancies. However, the dangerous childbirth idea was not Lawther's, but Dora Russell's, as she relates in her memoirs:

"I began to study official reports on the health and death rate of child-bearing women. ....We found that the average death rate of mothers was then four to five per thousand births. By contrast the death rate of miners from fatal accidents was 1.1 per thousand miners actually engaged in mining. Leah L'Estrange Malone and I than coined the slogan: 'It is four times as dangerous to bear a child as to work in a mine...'"[177]

Russell had stayed with Steve Lawther and his wife in 1926, while visiting the constituencies of Labour MPs who had voted against Ernest Thurtle's birth control advice Bill. The Lawthers sponsored Dora's meetings, and she recalls: "Their lodging was very simple. Mrs. Lawther, pregnant at that time, had to carry coals up several flights of stairs and cook on an open grate."[178] Life was indeed different for poor women.

Dora had made good use of her slogan about the dangers of childbearing, having already employed it to address the Independent Labour Party in 1924: "Making our usual plea based on the risks to life and health of child-bearing, I none the less added the comment that there seemed no reason for demanding an increasing population, nor could the Labour and Socialist programme of housing, education and endowment of motherhood be fundamentally carried out without reference to population growth."[179]

Espousing the aspirations of the Left, while warning that they cannot be achieved without population control, Russell demonstrates clearly how the left-wing birth control activists managed to be in the Labour Party, but not of it.

The theme of danger to women from childbearing was emphasised in a Workers' Birth Control Group memorandum to the Minister of Health in 1924

– but in this memo, it was the danger of illegal abortion caused, they alleged, by the refusal to allow women access to birth control knowledge. The memo included harrowing individual cases, and the assertion that the WBCG did not seek compulsory birth control. However, on the same page, Dr. Orr of Ealing Public Health Department insists:

"The reckless propagation of children by parents who are unable to give them reasonable nurture is a cause of great expense and a source of great weakness to the community."[180]   Once again, the mask had slipped, and the rhetoric of compassion slid inexorably into population control and eugenics. The Memorandum alleged that it was cruel to refuse contraceptive knowledge to women whose "…mental and physical health, and in many cases, environmental and economic circumstances, [made] it impossible for them to produce healthy children, still less to lead tolerable lives themselves."[181]

Wheatley had presumably been elected to try to make such lives more "tolerable", and to help the poor to have healthy children – not by encouraging them to restrict their families, but by promising better health care, a better environment, and better social security. In 1915, a collection of letters from poor mothers was published, *Maternity Letters from Working-women,* which made it plain where the needs of such mothers lay: "Skilled medical attention was particularly vital in the case of many of these women because of an almost universal lack of prenatal care." The average cost for a doctor to attend a confinement was about a guinea; for a midwife, ten to twelve shillings, and there was no maternity benefit.

'Letters' overwhelmingly mentions poverty as the cause of health problems. Almost every letter reiterates the lack of food, overwork before confinement, and excessively quick return to household chores after birth, as the prime causes of stillbirth and miscarriage, and often life long disablement for the mother. One woman whose husband earned 28 shillings a week, and who had seven children, three stillbirths and four miscarriages, wrote:

'I looked after my husband and children well, but I often went short of food myself, though my husband did not know it. He used to think that my appetite was bad and that I could not eat.'"[182] It was essential to keep husbands well fed, so that they were not laid up with sickness, with consequent lack of income. Conditions for women in those circumstances would be even more appalling. Many stinted their own food to ensure that the breadwinner was kept going.

The author's maternal grandmother was born at the end of the nineteenth century and lived in the East End of London. She had three stillborn children. Household chores were physically very demanding – fetching coals and water, washing and cleaning – all without labour-saving devices, or the servants that most birth control advocates kept. The focus of modern feminism tends to be on these women's lack of birth control but not, however, on their lack of indoor lavatories, vacuum cleaners, washing machines and sanitary towels.

Maternity Letters advocated a range of social improvements for poor mothers, but did not advocate contraceptive advice. Neither did the Labour Party's 'Protect the Nation's Mothers' in 1936. This booklet was deeply concerned with maternal deaths. It pointed out that there were variations in the maternal death rate (in general, higher in the North than the South). It was also high in certain industrial areas, such as Lancashire and Yorkshire, in certain mining areas, such as South Wales, and in sparsely populated areas, such as North Wales and Cumberland (thereby debunking a favourite Malthusian theory).

The authors quote a 1931 Report on Maternal Mortality by the Health Secretary of the League of Nations: "Puerperal fever (sepsis) leads to more deaths than any other complication of childbearing; but it is one of the causes which it is most easy to prevent by observing antiseptic principles, the favourable results of which have been strikingly demonstrated since their introduction." Indeed, puerperal sepsis – infection of the genital tract following childbirth - was the cause of 1,061 maternal deaths in 1933, or 40% of the total. Puerperal sepsis could follow either an abnormal birth where instruments had been used, where haemorrhage had occurred, or in a normal labour assisted by someone carrying the haemolytic streptococcus virus.[183] Insanitary living conditions, lack of piped water and lavatory facilities could mean that, while a normal confinement might pass without danger, any medical intervention would be likely to lead to deadly complications.

Were the birth controllers right, and would contraception - if poor women had wanted it, and if it had worked - have helped reduce the maternal mortality rate? 'Protect the Nation's Mothers' acknowledges that the maternal death rate was 3.87 per 1,000 live births in 1911, and that by 1933 it had risen to 4.51 maternal deaths per 1,000. But the number of births had fallen from 881,138 in 1911, to 580,413 in 1933. While stressing that measures should be taken to reduce the risks, and the need for better health care, housing and nutrition, the authors state: "The falling birth-rate means a larger proportion of first confinements, which are known to be the most dangerous. Therefore, it is sometimes argued, the high maternal death-rate is not so alarming as the figures might suggest."

Even with a falling overall birth rate, smaller families did not automatically make for safer motherhood. In fact, the focus on the maternal death rate resulted in a surprising discovery: it was actually *higher* for middle-class mothers than for working-class mothers.[184]

This provoked a public outcry. One possible explanation, according to Jane Lewis, was that the private nursing homes favoured by middle-class mothers were the most dangerous environment of all in which to give birth: "A case of sepsis would force the temporary closure of these institutions if reported, thus it was likely that either temperatures were not taken routinely, or that cases of sepsis were not reported and not isolated."[185]

Though maternal mortality rates remained a "stubborn problem"[186] during the Twenties and Thirties, motherhood was not the main killer of women of reproductive ages. Between 1921 and 1930, TB was by far the greatest killer, accounting for 26% of deaths of married women aged 15-44, whereas maternal mortality accounted for 17%. However, though absolute numbers were small, it was the only major cause of death to show an increase between the Wars.[187] Despite this, Russell and her colleagues continued to imply that poor women needed to limit their families for the sake of their health.

Of course, they had to include a call for better living conditions, but like all Malthusians they believed that, if poor families limited the numbers of their children, they would prosper, and there would be no need of social improvements. That is why Stella Browne toured the mining areas preaching birth control, during the 1920s.[188] Miners had always been noted for having large families, but during mid-Victorian years they lost nearly three of the 7.6 children born to them, leaving a net fertility of 4.6 — below that of most other occupational groups, including some of the middle classes.[189] Nevertheless, one of the Malthusians' obsessions was to help them curb their numbers by birth control. Like Stopes, they feared the revolutionary potential of starving hordes of discontented miners.

A 1929 Labour election pamphlet called maternal death rates a "disgrace to our civilisation", and repeated the idea of childbirth being four times as dangerous as working in the mines. However, it made no recommendations for contraception. It proposed instead to expand National Health Insurance for free medical and nursing care for women; introduce maternity leave for working mothers; give a cash maternity benefit; give free or cheap milk, food and educational services to mothers before and after childbirth; make 'home helps' available; introduce maternity homes, beds in hospitals, consultant services for pregnant women; better midwifery; convalescent homes for mothers and babies. In the 1920s, such things were unheard of luxuries for poor women.

Dismissing objections of exorbitant expense, the authors state: "Two capital ships for the Navy make as large a demand on the Budget as the services we propose. Yet maternal welfare is far more important than warships."

The ideas contained within the Election pamphlet were never to bear fruit. Mothers continued to suffer, so that Wal Hannington records, in the even greater poverty of the 1930s: "Many of the young in the Distressed Areas know only of a mother worn out by worry and fear of the future; a mother trying to provide meals each day and to keep the home going on an utterly inadequate income."[190] Giving evidence to the Birkett Committee on abortion, on behalf of the Union of Catholic Mothers, Dr Mary Cardwell stated that twenty working-class mothers chosen at random from her patients never had any butter, or expensive vegetables. They had only one pint of milk for the whole family, once a week on Sundays.[191]

The Distinguished and the Eminent

Jane Lewis, in *Politics of Motherhood*, gives an interesting interpretation of the birth control issue: "The falling birth rate and the high abortion rate alone show that women were anxious to control their own fertility, but they did not openly support the birth control cause until Marie Stopes provided a more respectable justification for the use of contraceptives during the 1920s".[192]

Apparently, women secretly approved of birth control, and longed to use it, but were only given the 'go ahead' by Marie Stopes. But Stopes' justifications for birth control use could hardly be termed "respectable", even when they were not frankly offensive.

Notwithstanding, the pioneers of birth control are frequently described by historians as 'distinguished' and 'eminent': "The eminent NBCC hierarchy served to enhance the cause of birth control.... An impressive array of thirty-four vice-presidents..." "Many early members shared with Eva Hubback a humanitarian interest in spreading the knowledge of birth control." (Leathard)[193] "Those women pioneers were a lively and intrepid group..."(Russell)[194] "During the next year or so, other distinguished names were added..."(Sargent Florence)[195] "...a courageous, brilliant band." (Jeger)[196]

Controversial figures within the birth control movement are given a sympathetic handling: "Rose Witcop and Guy Aldred, impressed by the amount of suffering caused to mothers through ignorance..."(Russell)[197] "She [Marie Stopes] hated to be thought of as an eccentric, and the phrase 'constructive birth control' was used by her to indicate that she was certainly not anti-baby or anti-child. She simply wanted to see mothers and children both happy and healthy".[198] "However much they [Sanger and Stopes] may have been motivated by high ideals and humanitarian principles, each tended to regard birth control and its advocacy as her own personal property. Both ladies were fond of publicity..." (Wood/Suitters)[199] "...Marie Carmichael Stopes, an eloquent and impassioned [birth control] advocate".[200] "Marie Stopes's courageous denunciation of the unplanned family which spelt poverty and misery to the children, and ill-health and unhappiness to the mother..."(Summerskill)[201]

Stocks waxes eloquent: "...Marie Stopes, the Mrs. Pankhurst of the birth-control movement, broke the silence barrier which shrouded that subject with a reverberating supersonic bang"[202] and still more eloquent: "I think that her desire to work in her own way on her own lines...was connected with a belief...that she was directly inspired by God...Joan of Arc was so inspired after her triumph at Orleans...The attitude of Gladys Aylward...is in many ways comparable to that of St Joan...I am glad to have known Marie Stopes and Gladys Aylward, and wish I could have known Joan of Arc".[203]

Meanwhile, Potts and Selman state: "...[Malthus] was moved by the sufferings of the poor..."[204]

The Malthusian movement is blamed for putting off people from contraception, but criticism of their offensive ideology is muted: "Women's groups did not make any formal demand for birth control until the 1920s. This was because the birth control movement had been dominated by the Malthusian League up to World War I, and the league's philosophy did not inspire public support."[205] "The league's academic tone and dismal philosophy were unattractive."(Lewis)[206] "The neo-Malthusians…had a special interest in the benefits of population control and economics…" (Leathard)[207] "…the Malthusian League, which propagandised population control as the answer to poverty."(Shapiro)[208] "…the Malthusian League, which believed that overpopulation was the cause of poverty…"(Seal)[209] "…there was, as the League's 1912 annual report put it, a crying need for a propaganda campaign among the poorest classes…"(Fryer)[210]

Leathard, Shapiro, Seal, Fryer, Russell, Sargent Florence, Jeger, Wood and Suitters, Blacker, Summerskill, Stocks, Fryer, Potts and Selman, have all been involved in the campaign for fertility control.

The refusal of feminism to hitch its star to the wagon of birth control is treated as an annoying puzzle. Joseph and Olive Banks, in *Feminism and Family Planning in Victorian England*, give the impression that the feminist movement did not get involved in the birth control issue because they were 'anti sex'. Nevertheless, feminism is conscripted in order to place in a sympathetic light even those who would have made the worst ambassadresses of feminism: "Malthusian League members, Mrs. How-Martyn and Mrs. Bessie Drysdale and clinic pioneer, Marie Stopes, were amongst the vigorous birth control campaigners who had worked for the suffrage. They were to be joined by many others". (Leathard)[211]

Summing up the early birth control movement, Leathard enthuses: "It was a movement for social justice: the clinic was the chosen device to enable poorer mothers to receive medical advice and instruction. It was a poverty crusade to rescue lower-class families from ignorance and squalor through the rational control of fertility. It was a feminist crusade, pioneered by women, to rescue wives from male selfishness." She continues, somewhat abruptly: "It was the means, as some pioneers saw it, to achieve population control and to check inferior racial stock". Quickly recovering from this admission, she ends with a flourish: "United in the rightness of their cause, though later divided on certain issues, birth controllers faced almost total opposition from the churches, the medical profession and by most of the respectable world. Thus animated and defiant, the clinic pioneers came together inspired by varying beliefs".[212]

The birth controllers may have had "varying beliefs", but most had one thing in common. It was money. Lady Denman was the daughter of Lord Cowdray, who had "amassed vast wealth" during his career. She "contributed generously to the cause".[213] The Drysdales financed the Malthusian League largely from their own pockets.[214] Both Stopes and Margaret Sanger had married rich second husbands who generously financed their wives' endeavours in the birth control field.[215] Janet Chance's husband was a wealthy investment banker.[216] Lady Astor was an American millionairess, a member of the 'Cliveden

Set'.[217] Mary (later Lady) Stocks was one of the many middle-class women who worked in the birth control movement, and founded and ran the clinics. She and the other birth control pioneers all kept servants.[218]

Some birth control activists, as we have seen, used the rhetoric of socialism, while retaining   middle-class lifestyles and attitudes. The effort involved in trying to keep two hats on one head led to some strange value judgements about those who refused to support their cause. Russell, for example, hints that Ramsay MacDonald's "liking for upper-class society" was "weakening his drive towards true socialism."[219] She recalls - in between descriptions of dinner parties in Chelsea - preparing herself carefully for the Labour Party Conference where she was due to speak: "I dressed for the occasion in a scarlet jersey long-waisted dress with a short cape tied at the throat with dark blue braid to give myself confidence".[220] Despite complaining of poverty, she was able to keep servants.

However, even wealthy women were forced to raise money for birth control. Dr Edith Summerskill and Frida Laski organised a fund-raising 'Malthusian Ball' at the Dorchester Hotel in 1933, "to which Princess Alice, Countess of Athlone, and a great many other titled persons gave their patronage".

The skimming over of the beliefs and propaganda of the birth controllers, leads to the supposition that they were at best misunderstood, and at worst, that they were simply rather dotty – English eccentrics in the best tradition.[221]

Vivien Seal's description of the Malthusian League's clinic in East Street, Bermondsey, London, is an example of this confusion. She says it was "a great success". This is extraordinary in itself.[222] However, she adds: "Women and staff met opposition from the Catholic Church and were pelted with eggs, stones and apples. Windows were smashed and the walls daubed with graffiti such as 'whores'."[223] This makes it unclear whether the attacks were committed by the Catholic Church or others. In fact feminists – and, indeed, anyone brave or foolish enough to stand on a soapbox – was liable to be pelted in those days, but not necessarily by religious opponents.[224]

Some birth control advocates may have had good motives. Some had exceedingly dubious motives. But their treatment in the vast majority of histories is dangerously misleading. Everyone has their own favourite historical figures; it is understandable that their reputations are treated more gently than those for whom we feel little sympathy. But it is extraordinary to read of characters like Casanova, or the Marquis de Sade, who made a career out of abusing women and children, treated so unjudgementally – especially when speaking of a subject overwhelmingly deemed to be a 'woman's' issue. We are forced to ask why such people's reputations have been glossed over.

We return briefly to Charles Bradlaugh, and his beliefs, here expressed in his "Labour's Prayer":

"Yet all the prayers that labour ever uttered since the first breath of human life, have not availed so much for human happiness as will the earnest examination by one generation of this, the greatest of all social questions, the root of all political problems, the foundation of all civil progress".

For Bradlaugh and his fellow birth control advocates, the greatest of all social questions was population, and it was people who were the root of all problems.

NOTES

[1] By 1905, George Drysdale's *Physical, Sexual and Natural Religion*, (later titled *Elements of Social Science*), had sold 88,000 copies, and had been translated into ten European languages. (*The Birth Controllers*, p110) Within three months of their arrest, Bradlaugh and Besant sold 125,000 copies of *Fruits of Philosophy*, trebling the sales of the previous forty-three years. They sold another 185,000 copies by the end of the decade. (*Birth Control and the Population Question in England 1877-1930*, p326) By the time Annie Besant's conversion to theosophy made her withdraw her *Laws of Population*, priced at 6d, it had sold 175,000 copies.

[2] *Birth Control and the Population Question in England 1877-1930, op cit*, p326.

[3] *The Birth Controllers, op cit*, p185

[4] *The Birth Controllers, op cit*, p179 and 311n.

[5] *Society and Fertility, op cit*, p290.

[6] He complained to Marie Stopes about birth control campaigners. (Rev B H Streeter to Stopes, 15 November 1919, 24 January, 7 February, 27 September 1920, Add. MSS. 58554, in *Birth Control and the Population Question in England 1877-1930, p240.*

[7] 'Bad tidings of great joy', Joanna Trevelyan, *Guardian*, 21.6.1994

[8] *The Birth Controllers, op cit*, p177.

[9] "There can be no doubt that the success of this movement [Malthusianism] resulted from the fact that, as compared with the period before 1870, a sufficiently large section of the public was eager for information on the subject. This does not mean that the public taboo was raised from discussions of contraception."(*Feminism and Family Planning in Victorian England*, p91); See also *The Birth Controllers*, p165 – Besant's *Laws of Population*, which she published after the obscenity trial against *Fruits of Philosophy*, was *never* prosecuted.

[10] See *Feminism and Family Planning in Victorian England, op cit.*

[11] *History of the Condom*, leaflet, LRC Products Ltd., North Circular Road, London E4

[12] *Marie Stopes: a biography, op cit*, p315. Blacker was reporting on the Family Planning Association clinics for the years 1938-1947, apparently not taking account of the fact that many women were separated from their husbands during those years.

[13] According to Himes, no figures were available for the numbers manufactured in England and Germany. (*Medical History of Contraception*, p201) Audrey Donnithorne, in her 1958 study of the British rubber manufacturing industry, does not mention condom production. (*British Rubber Manufacturing: An Economic Study of Innovations*, Gerald Duckworth & Co Ltd., London)

[14] "approximately one in five servicemen was infected with gonorrhoea" (*Birth Control and the Population Question in England 1877-1930, p170.*

[15] See Sheila Jeffreys, *The Spinster and Her Enemies: Feminism and Sexuality 1880-1930*, Pandora, 1985.

[16] *Family Limitation*, pp19-20, 1925 Edition.

[17] *op cit*, pp18-19.

[18] *op cit, p16.*

[19] *op cit,* pp16-17.

[20] "'There is very little evidence to suggest that even after the first world war contraceptive devices were widely used by the working class. Few knew about them; many could not afford them." (*A Woman's Place*, p97). See also Anne Smith, *Women Remember: An Oral History*, Routledge, 1989.

[21] See *Sex, Politics & Society, op cit*

[22] See *Genesis*

[23] *Sex and Destiny, op cit*, Chapter Five.

[24] *ibid* p109

[25] *A Woman's Place, op cit*, p95.

[26] In small houses, husbands sometimes slept in their sons' room, and wives in their daughters, in order to avoid the problem of growing children of both sexes sharing a bedroom - and sometimes to avoid further pregnancies. (*ibid*, p96)

[27] *ibid*, p99

[28] First published 1792; taken from the Penguin edition, 1985, p315.

[29] The records of birth control clinics were, as we have seen, inaccurate, tending to inflate their successes, and ignore or excuse their failures; also, they depended on a small number of women, the location of the clinic, and the fact that those availing themselves of the facilities were already to some extent converted to the idea of family limitation. Records would not have covered those women whose husbands took responsibility for contraception, and those who objected to it for cultural or religious reasons.

[30] Elizabeth Roberts writes: "What information was available was obtained from the peer group, work-mates, friends and relations, including husbands and neighbours, although, as will be seen later, it would be unwise to over-emphasise the importance of the textile mill as a source of contraceptive advice." She goes on: "No respondent mentioned the Marie Stopes clinics or publications." (*A Woman's Place, op cit*, p95)

[31] See *The Birth Controllers, op cit*, pp24 & p32.

[32] F. Grose, *Guide*, 1796, in *Medical History of Contraception*, p200.

[33] See Peter Hitchens, *The Abolition of Britain, op cit*, for a useful overview of the drastic change in outlook of the British people, largely influenced by the advent of the contraceptive pill in the 1960s.

[34] "Why was contraception not more frequently resorted to by preliterate peoples? The widespread adoption of abortion and more especially of infanticide filled the need. These checks are immediate, practicable and certainly effective." (Himes, *Medical History of Contraception*, pp51-2)

[35] See also Draper, *Birth Control in the Modern World*; Fryer, *The Birth Controllers*; Potts and Selman, *Society and Fertility*; Diggory, Potts and Peel, *Abortion*, Cambridge University Press, 1977; Wood and Suitters, *The Fight for Acceptance: A History of Contraception*.

[36] *Medical History of Contraception, op cit*, p51-2

[37] Linda Gordon, *Women's Body, Woman's Right: Birth Control in America*, Penguin, 1990, p33.

[38] There is also the possibility that the 'illegitimate' child of a rival might be killed at the behest of a legal wife, in order to protect the inheritance of her own children.

[39] Napoleon Chagnon, *Yanomamo: The Fierce People*, New York, 1977, in *Sex and Destiny*, p188.

[40] *Sex and Destiny*, p189.

[41] *ibid,* pp190-191

[42] In 2000, 70 million men aged 25-49 were forced to remain bachelors; in 1999, police investigated 19,000 cases of women sold as wives against their will, while more than 60,000 people were involved in trafficking of brides. (*Catholic Times,* 7.11.1999)

[43] In Sparta, in early times, sacrifices were made to Ares, the god of war (or spirit of battle) from among prisoners of war. (Interestingly enough, this aspect of killing is not mentioned as a 'population control' method by birth control historians.)

[44] J.D.J. Havard, 'A Bounty on Infanticide', *New Society,* 11.6.1964.

[45] Emmeline Pankhurst, *My own story,* Virago Ltd., London, 1979, pp27-8. First published Hearst's International Library Co., Inc. USA, 1914.

[46] In more recent years, persistently high numbers of cot deaths gave the opportunity again to allege that secret infanticide was being practised; however, since government advice to lay infants on their backs was reversed, the number of such deaths has been reduced, once again pointing to environmental factors.

[47] *New Generation,* November 1923, pp128-9.

[48] Cover notes, *Medical History of Contraception.*

[49] Cover notes, *The Fight for Acceptance.*

[50] FPA Annual Report, 1992-3.

[51] Cover notes, *Birth Control in the Modern World.*

[52] Phillips, A, Rakusen, J., (Eds.), *Our Bodies Ourselves: A Health Book by and for Women,* Penguin Books, 1986, p.236

[53] See Appendix I for details of birth control groups.

[54] For more information, see *The Fight for Family Planning; The Birth Controllers; Birth Control and the Population Question in England 1877-1930.*

[55] See Appendix I.

[56] See: *Marie Stopes: a biography;* Lella Sargent Florence, *Progress Report on Birth Control,* Heinneman, 1956; *Birth Control in the Modern World; The Fight for Acceptance; Marie Stopes, Eugenics and the English Birth Control Movement.*

[57] After 1928, when full suffrage was achieved, NUSEC split into two wings; the NCEC pressed for further equal rights legislation, and the Union of Townswomen's Guilds, which modelled themselves on the Women's Institutes, concentrated on education.

[58] See *The Fight for Family Planning; The Birth Controllers; Progress Report on Birth Control;* Mary Stocks, *My Commonplace Book,* Peter Davies, London 1970; *The Spinster and Her Enemies; Birth Control and the Population Question in England 1877-1930.*

[59] See *The Fight for Family Planning.*

[60] *The Fight for Family Planning; The Fight for Acceptance; Birth Control in the Modern World.*

[61] *The Fight for Family Planning, op cit.*

[62] SPBCC clinics (Walworth Women's Welfare Centre) Annual Report 1931-32.

[63] *A New World for Women, op cit,* p51.

[64] *The New Generation,* II, 1 (1923) p1, in *The Fight for Family Planning,* p28.

[65] See *The Birth Controllers; A New World for Women; Birth Control and the Population Question in England 1877-1930; Marie Stopes: a biography.*

[66] *Birth Control and the Population Question in England 1877-1930, op cit,* p302.

[67] *ibid p282*

[68] *New Generation*, October 1924, p111, in *Birth Control and the Population Question in England 1877-1930*, p302.

[69] *New Generation*, January 1937.

[70] See *The Birth Controllers*, p237: "…antagonism and suspicion gave place to sympathy and interest when the audience 'found that we wanted nothing from them, and were supported by no party'. (Drysdale, 'Neo-Malthusianism in South London', in *The Malthusian*, 15 May 1921)

[71] *Birth Control and the Population Question in England 1877-1930, op cit*, p84.

[72] *ibid* p80

[73] 13.1.1924, in *Control of Life, op cit*, p94.

[74] 18.3.1932, in *ibid* p95.

[75] Under the headline "LORD DAWSON MUST GO", the *Sunday Express* attacked the King's Physician for supporting birth control, "wearing the grimy mantle of Malthas (sic)," 16th October 1921.

[76] See *The Birth Controllers, op cit*.

[77] R. Dowse and J. Peel, 'The Politics of Birth Control', *Political Studies*, XIII, 2, 1965, p184, in *The Fight for Family Planning*, p29.

[78] *The Fight for Family Planning, op cit*, p29.

[79] Dora Russell, *The Tamarisk Tree: Vol.1, My Quest for Liberty and Love*, Virago, 1977.

[80] See Greta Jones, *Social Hygiene in Twentieth Century Britain*, Croom Helm, London, 1986.

[81] For Dalton's racist views, see Andrew Roberts, *Eminent Churchillians*, Phoenix, 1994, p215

[82] FPA, EC Minutes, 30 June 1944, 28 November 1944, in *The Fight for Family Planning*, p72.

[83] *The Tamarisk Tree, op cit*, p153.

[84] Ledbetter, *A History of the Malthusian League 1877-1927*, in *Birth Control and the Population Question in England 1877-1930*, p154.

[85] Croom Helm, London, 1980, p200.

[86] *Birth Control and the Population Question in England 1877-1930, op cit*, p56.

[87] *ibid* p178.

[88] Annie Besant, *Nethercot*, pp242-74; *Malthusian*, November 1889, p85, in *Birth Control and the Population Question in England 1877-1930*, p87.

[89] *Malthusian*, May 1879; January 1885; July 1891, in *Birth Control and the Population Question in England 1877-1930*, pp74-75.

[90] *Malthusian*, July 1879, and February 1887, in *ibid*, p76.

[91] *Birth Control and the Population Question in England 1877-1930*, p79.

[92] 15 February and 15 March 1919.

[93] *Malthusian*, October 1915, in *Birth Control and the Population Question in England 1877-1930*, p88.

[94] See *A New World for Women, op cit*.

[95] *Birth Control and the Population Question in England 1877-1930, op cit*, p192.

[96] "He, She and It", by Bessie I. Drysdale, in *New Generation*, January 1922. (Drysdale does not reveal whether this short story is based on her own home life.)

[97] *Birth Control and the Population Question in England 1877-1930, op cit, p286*.

[98] See *The Fight for Acceptance*, p135, for attempts to convert an unnamed charity worker to spreading birth control amongst the poor: "One package of leaflets had quite the opposite effect.

It was delivered to a lady who was well known for her welfare work among the poor, and who was noted for showing great bravery during the Peterloo 'massacre' of 1819. The receipt of the package seems to have given her a shock, and she took some trouble to try to discover the origin of the leaflets. She imagined the papers to be part of a plot to discredit her, and that they must have been issued by the followers of Malthus. She wrote to the Attorney-General about the matter but no prosecutions followed."

[99] A voluntary commission of enquiry into the falling birth rate, held 1913-1916.

[100] NCPM, 'Declining Birth-Rate', in *Birth Control and the Population Question in England 1877-1930*, p126.

[101] *ibid* p127.

[102] *Laws of Population*, in *The Birth Controllers*, p165.

[103] *The Tamarisk Tree, op cit.*

[104] The petition asked that "institutions under the control of the Ministry should give birth control advice to mothers who desired it, and that doctors in welfare centres should be allowed to give such advice when they considered it medically advisable." (*The Tamarisk Tree*, p171)

[105] See *Birth Control and the Population Question in England 1877-1930; The Fight for Family Planning; Politics of Motherhood; The Tamarisk Tree; Abortion in England 1900-1967.*

[106] Julian Symons, *The General Strike: A historical portrait*, Readers Union, The Cresset Press, London, 1959.

[107] *The Tamarisk Tree, op cit*, p171.

[108] *The Fight for Family Planning, op cit*, p29.

[109] *The Birth Controllers, op cit*, p259.

[110] *Politics of Motherhood, op cit*, p198.

[111] *Abortion in England 1900-1967, op cit*, p86.

[112] *Birth Control and the Population Question in England 1877-1930, op cit, p289.*

[113] D. Russell to Stopes, 31 March, 4, 8 April 1924, Stopes Papers, Add. MSS. 58556.

[114] *New Generation*, April 1922, in *Birth Control and the Population Question in England 1877-1930*, p194.

[115] *The Tamarisk Tree, op cit*, p172.

[116] *ibid* p171.

[117] The Labour Party Reports, 1925-27, p231.

[118] *ibid*, p232

[119] *ibid*, p233

[120] SA/ALR Box 53.

[121] *Birth Control and the Population Question in England 1877-1930, op cit* p284.

[122] *The Tamarisk Tree, op cit*, p172.

[123] *ibid* p70.

[124] *ibid* p179.

[125] *New Generation*, November 1923, p134.

[126] Dorothy Jewson, 'The Labour Party Conference and Birth Control', *The New Generation*, November 1925, p123 and p127.

[127] *New Generation*, January 1937.

[128] *Birth Control and the Population Question in England 1877-1930, op cit, p178.*

[129] *ibid* p285

[130] *The Tamarisk Tree, op cit*, p173. See also *Abortion in England 1900-1967*, p86: "The title was purposely chosen to prevent association with Malthusian or eugenic ideas."

[131] *Birth Control News*, July 1924, in *Birth Control and the Population Question in England 1877-1930*, p286.

[132] *The Fight for Family Planning, op cit*, pp29-30.

[133] *ibid* p32.

[134] *Birth Control and the Population Question in England 1877-1930, op cit, p286.*

[135] *The Tamarisk Tree, op cit*, p174.

[136] *ibid* p183.

[137] Russell and Dorothy Thurtle agreed that the Executive Committee of the Labour Party accepted women "so long as they have no opinions of their own and are willing to do the donkey work of the Party". (Dora Russell, *Hypatia*, p7, in *Abortion in England 1900-1967*, p87); "Complaints [were made] about male insensitivity or indifference to the needs and aspirations of women workers". (*Birth Control and the Population Question in England 1877-1930*, p286)

[138] *The Tamarisk Tree, op cit*, p70.

[139] *ibid*

[140] Guy Aldred, *No Traitor's Gait*, in *A New World for Women*, p23.

[141] *Abortion in England 1900-1967l, op cit*, p86.

[142] *The Tamarisk Tree, op cit*, p70.

[143] *ibid* p185.

[144] Witcop to Sanger, 12 May, 1 July 1925, Sanger Papers, Carton 21, in *Birth Control and the Population Question in England 1877-1930*, p301.

[145] *Birth Control and the Population Question in England 1877-1930, op cit, p290.*

[146] 'Report of the…Conference of the Labour Party (1927).

[147] *ibid* p232.

[148] *A New World for Women, op cit*, p39.

[149] *ibid* p54.

[150] *ibid* p57.

[151] *Birth Control and the Population Question in England 1877-1930, op cit*, p296.

[152] *Labour Woman*, in *Birth Control and the Population Question in England 1877-1930*, pp284-5.

[153] D. Russell to Stopes, 2 October 1929, Stopes Papers, Add.MSS. 58556, in *Birth Control and the Population Question in England 1877-1930*, pp296-7. (Soloway's comment that Phillips was unmarried, is hardly relevant; so were many of the birth control activists, including Cicely Hamilton and Stella Browne; so were many of the feminists whose lack of wedded bliss did not exclude them from the struggle for the vote.

[154] The Labour party executive committee tried to exclude any discussion of birth control from the agenda, taking advantage of the fact that the previous Labour Women's Conference, interrupted by the General Strike, had not been able to vote on the matter, despite receiving sixty resolutions advocating birth control 'on the rates'. (*Birth Control and the Population Question in England 1877-1930*, p294)

[155] *Report of the Conference of the Labour Party*, (1926), in *Birth Control and the Population Question in England 1877-1930*, p295.

[156] *ibid*

[157] *Fifty Years March: The Rise of the Labour Party*, Odhams Press Ltd, London

[158] Vol. III, p52-3.

[159] *Birth Control and the Population Question in England 1877-1930, op cit, p287.*

[160] *ibid*; see also *A New World for Women*, p56.

[161] *The Tamarisk Tree, op cit*, p189.

[162] *ibid* pp190-191

[163] *ibid* pp189-90

[164] *Report of the Conference of the Labour Party*, (1926), in *Birth Control and the Population Question in England 1877-1930*, p295.

[165] *A New World for Women, op cit*, p58; see also Sheila Jeffreys, *The Spinster and Her Enemies*, which traces the decline of organised feminism under the influence of eugenics.

[166] Memorandum from the North-Western Federation of Societies for Equal Citizenship, MH71/24, PRO, in *Abortion in England 1900-1967*, p114

[167] See *Birth Control and the Population Question in England 1877-1930*; *The Birth Controllers*; *The Fight for Family Planning, Politics of Motherhood.*

[168] See *Birth Control and the Population Question in England 1877-1930*; *The Birth Controllers*; *The Fight for Family Planning, Politics of Motherhood.*

[169] *The Tamarisk Tree, op cit*, p170.

[170] *ibid* p43 and p36.

[171] See *Hidden from History: 300 Years of Women's Oppression and the Fight Against It.*

[172] *The Fight for Family Planning, op cit*, p55

[173] *ibid*

[174] *ibid*

[175] *The Birth Controllers, op cit*, p260.

[176] Labour Party Conference Report, 1927.

[177] *The Tamarisk Tree, op cit*, p171.

[178] *ibid*, p183

[179] *ibid*, p177

[180] Memorandum on Birth Control presented to the Minister of Health by the Workers' Birth Control Group, May 9th 1924, p7.

[181] *ibid*, p3

[182] *Maternity: Letters from Working-women, collected by the Women's Co-operative Guild*, ed. Margaret Llewelyn Davies, G. Bell & Sons Ltd., 1915 (new introduction, Virago edition, 1978).

[183] *Politics of Motherhood, op cit*, p122.

[184] Mortality rates for the years 1930-32 from pregnancy and childbearing per 1,000 live births were calculated for the wives in men of different social groups, based on occupational classifications obtaining at the Census of 1931. For all married women the rate was 4.13; for wives of men in professional and allied occupations, it was 4.44; for wives of skilled and semi-skilled workers, it was about average; for wives of unskilled workers, it was 3.89. (*Times*, 18.11.36)

[185] Jellett, *The Cause and Prevention of Mat. Mort.*, p124, in Politics of Motherhood, p134.

[186] The Maternal Mortality Committee, 1930, in Politics of Motherhood, p117.

[187] *Politics of Motherhood, op. cit*, p182.

[188] "At her urging the league began concentrating most of its limited resources on working-class organisations, and in the summer of 1923 she led a mission to the Rhondda valley to preach birth control to the distressed miners." (*Birth Control and the Population Question 1877-1930*, p197)

[189] *ibid* p43

[190] Wal Hannington, *The Problem of the Distressed Areas*, Victor Gollancz Ltd., London, 1937, p78.

[191] MH71/24 AC Paper No.72, Memo from National Committee of the Union of Catholic Mothers, presented by Mary G. Cardwell MD, December 1937.

[192] Croom Helm, London, pp196-7.

[193] *The Fight for Family Planning, op cit*, p44-5.

[194] *The Tamarisk Tree, op cit*, p173.

[195] Lela Sargent Florence, describing the Birmingham Clinic Executive Council. (*Progress Report on Birth Control*, p254)

[196] L. Jeger, 'The Politics of Family Planning', *Political Quarterly*, 33, 1 (1962) p51, in *The Fight for Family Planning*, p45.

[197] Dora Russell, in *The Encyclopaedia of the Labour Movement*, Vol.1, Caxton, London, ed. H. B. Lees-Smith.

[198] *The Fight for Acceptance, op cit*, p163.

[199] *ibid* p180

[200] C P Blacker, *Eugenics: Galton and After*, Gerald Duckworth, London, 1952.

[201] Edith Summerskill, *A Woman's World*, Heinnemann, London, 1967, p55.

[202] *My Commonplace Book*, op cit, p124.

[203] Mary Stocks, *Still More Commonplace*, Peter Davies, London, 1973, p22.

[204] *Sex and Fertility, op cit*, p291.

[205] *Politics of Motherhood*, op cit.

[206] *ibid*

[207] *The Fight for Family Planning, op cit*, p6.

[208] *Contraception: A Practical and Political Guide*, Rose Shapiro, Virago, 1987, p4.

[209] Vivien Seal, *Whose Choice? Working Class Women and the Control of Fertility*, Fortress Books, 1990.

[210] *The Birth Controllers, op cit*, p236.

[211] *The Fight for Family Planning, op cit*, p9.

[212] *ibid* p10

[213] *ibid* p45

[214] See *Birth Control and the Population Question in England 1877-1930, op cit.*

[215] See *The Fight for Acceptance, op cit*, p164.

[216] *Birth Control and the Population Question in England 1877-1930, op cit, p88.*

[217] See *My Commonplace Book*, op cit.

[218] *ibid*

[219] *The Tamarisk Tree, op cit*, p179.

[220] *ibid* p172

[221] My father was fond of saying that if you had money, you were considered eccentric – if not, you were just mad.

[222] Only two women attended in November 1921, and eight in January 1922. However, in January 1923, attendance was claimed at 258 – but this may have had something to do with other classes, including sewing, which they added to "little homely birth control talks". (Report of 5th International Neo-Malthusian and Birth Control Conference, in *The Birth Controllers,* pp251-2)

[223] *ibid*

[224] See Barbara Winslow, *Sylvia Pankhurst: Sexual Politics and Political Activism*, UCL Press, 1996: "It was not an easy or pleasant task because, although many women attended the meetings, more often than not young boys would show up at the outdoor gatherings and throw garbage, dead fish and newspapers soaked in urine." (p34) "The rally was almost spoiled when some young boys attempted to heckle and throw stones and garbage at Pankhurst. The police stood by and refused to help the demonstraters, but the women were protected by the large number of dockers who came on the demonstration." (p46)

Chapter Four

THE ROOT OF ALL EVIL

Persuasion and coercion; the 'perfect contraceptive'; abortion as birth control; the puzzle of birth control; fear of the poor.

Jeremy Bentham (1748-1832), political economist and birth control advocate, developed a system of ethics called 'utilitarianism'. Briefly, this means testing any law, rule, or action, by its utility, or consequences – whether it will bring about the greatest happiness of the greatest number of people. This had distinct appeal in an age where the mass of people were ruled by a tiny elite. However, in a democracy, it can mean that minorities, and the weakest, may suffer from the demands of those in the majority - the strongest.[1] It depends also on how you interpret 'happiness'; indeed, how you interpret 'people'.

Though seemingly innocuous and acceptable to all, Bentham's rule was open to misinterpretation and abuse, as J.S. Mill foresaw. Predicting the consequences of any law before it is passed is not an exact science either, though our 'prophets' were frequently confident enough to do so.

Utilitarian arguments were used by the tiny minority involved in the birth control campaign. This minority, with strong opinions on a single issue, and employing the rhetoric of compassion, eventually succeeded in winning public funds (supplied by the majority) for their plan to control the reproduction of that majority. They succeeded partly by representing *themselves* as the majority, interpreting – in the absence of any clear evidence – silence, or even outright denial, that this was what the majority desired.

After a brief, unsuccessful flirtation with compulsory birth control, they emphasised the voluntary nature of their schemes. Its advocates claimed that birth control needed to be provided, because that was what people wanted, but then puzzled over the perennial problem of birth control. Once it had been provided, those who were said to need it most, did not use it. Potts and Selman remark: "The continued existence of large unplanned families in the poorer sections of many developed societies.... has led to many studies of the relationship between fertility and poverty. There has been dispute about the extent to which the poor have more children because they want more. Some writers...argue that this is a major factor, while others have seen the differences as largely due to unwanted births and a lack of realistic opportunities to plan their families."[2]

Though the poor continued to have more children, they didn't – according to birth control experts - really want them. The fact that the poor do not take up opportunities for family planning when they are available is somehow overlooked.

Excuses are found for this lack of response, while the fact that other, more practical relief for families is quickly claimed, is ignored.[3] Unlike Marie Antoinette, who at least, so it is said, allowed the poor the opportunity to eat cake when they had no bread, birth controllers offered neither bread nor cake, but endlessly studied the poor's lack of enthusiasm for having fewer children. These studies found them to be 'ignorant'.[4] They were oppressed in their family relationships.[5] They were 'timid'.[6] They were 'superstitious'.[7] They were under religious edict.[8] They lacked 'motivation'.[9]

It was found that "...government propaganda and positive measures of assistance to induce people to undertake family planning in several parts of the world...[were] only partially successful..."[10] Garrett Hardin describes the attitude of birth control campaigners in the 1960s: "...they claim that satisfactory motivation is shown by the popular desire (shown by opinion surveys in all countries) to have the means of family limitation, and that therefore the problem is one of inventing and distributing the best possible contraceptive devices."[11] But, as Elizabeth Draper laments: "...there remain some big questions to be answered. How far are present methods used, and if nothing better is found is it possible to 'get them across' to all users? Even with perfect methods, would it still be necessary to 'get them across'?"[12]

Opinion surveys may have discovered a 'vast, unmet need' for contraception,[13] and they have certainly been useful in boosting demands for more funds for birth control. The problem with such surveys is that (as many doorstep canvassers have found during election campaigns) the quickest way to get rid of such questioners is to answer 'yes' to every question.

All population control advocates have claimed that they want people to use birth control because of the benefits it will bring to individuals, couples, and families – even to children. They would have little success, after all, if they told people that they should use something that would have a negative impact on their lives, for the sake of the happiness of the greatest number. Keeping a balance between voluntary and compulsory birth control has meant that its advocates have veered between exhortations and threats. The resultant arguments are a strange mix of compassion, human rights and individual fulfilment, combined with threats and warnings of the need to bring down population growth.

Kingsley Davis called 'family planning' a "euphemism for contraception". He was honest enough to admit: "One suspects that the entire question of [population] goals is instinctively left vague because thorough limitation of population growth would run counter to national and group aspirations." A real population control programme, he says, would mean "deliberate influence over all attributes of a population, including its age-sex structure, geographical distribution, racial composition, genetic quality, and total size."[14]

This is the problem that family planners face. Population control is just that. It cannot be achieved voluntarily. The rhetoric of family planning says that making birth control available gives women the choice of how many children to have, but Davis demands: "...suppose a woman does not want to use any contraceptive until after she has had four children. This is the type of question that is seldom raised in the family-planning literature."[15]

The aims of population control and family planning inevitably conflict. However, since the vast majority of population control advocates support 'family planning', we must presume that somehow, such programmes do serve the purposes of population control. But whether they are called population control or family planning, these programmes eventually collide with the age-old problem of how to make people do something they don't want to do.

The Malthusian priests saw the guardians of women's virtue – Church and State - as stumbling blocks to the spread of their gospel of birth control. Once those obstacles had been largely removed, there was yet another obstacle – women's reluctance to use birth control. The wheel had turned full circle. Once again women's sensibilities were proving difficult.

Population control advocates Joseph and Olive Banks realised, in 1965, that it was no good relying on a feminist approach to family planning. It was male influence that was vital in getting women to control their fertility, and they discussed ways of reaching wives through their husbands. The Bankses perceived the purpose of family planning as a device to bring down population growth, but they, too, acknowledged a serious problem: "Female modesty inculcated early in childhood makes many women reluctant to bring up such matters..."[16]

This anxiety is echoed by Edwin Brooks in 1973. Brooks, who as a Labour MP introduced the National Health Service (Family Planning) Bill of 1967, saw "uncontrolled parenthood" as "a very real malady". While claiming to want to give women choice, he drew attention to the Family Planning Association's difficulties in promoting family planning in Asian communities, arising from the problem of "the extreme modesty of Asian women".[17]

Kingsley Davis, writing in 1964, concurs: "The problem woman, from the standpoint of family planners, is the one who wants 'as many as come', or 'as many as God sends'."[18]

Such female reluctance was not only seen as a problem in poor countries. Having repeatedly called for freely available contraceptives, so that those who needed them most would at last be able to use them, it must have proved disappointing that some British women were still having more children than they should. Leathard calls this the "problem of the indifferent contraceptor": "Ignorance about methods, mistaken anxiety about the dangers, genuine dislike for the most efficient methods – sheath, cap and pill – the need for prescriptions and fittings, the inconvenience and 'medical atmosphere' of local family planning clinics, all combined to make a proportion of married women indifferent contraceptors."[19]

The next logical step in the process was to change people's (especially women's) attitudes to contraception by advertising. In 1970, a Report prepared by the Research Department of the Labour Party for the Labour Party Women's Conference called for the: "...establishment of a comprehensive family planning service under the NHS...backed by a substantial advertising campaign on the facilities available (and on the gravity of the population problem)..."[20]

In 1972, the Birth Control Campaign also called for more publicity for 'family planning' to "reduce the rate of increase of the population": "The importance of expenditure on publicity and advertising on a large scale...should not be forgotten." It was not until 2001, however, that condoms were advertised on London bus shelters – but by 2001, the over-the-counter supply of the morning-after pill was being openly promoted by pharmacies.

Realising – perhaps from experience of the 1930 edict - that simply legislating for something to be made permissible was not enough, the 1972 BCC plan also proposed a "Special Unit...with powers to visit any area and make recommendations concerning its birth control provision." This was defined in the Report as "comprehensive fertility control" – contraception, sterilisation and abortion. Since the success of the plan would need to be judged on its objective - the falling birth rate – this, presumably, was where the Special Unit would play a part.[21]

Oblique references to "low contraceptive prevalence"[22] and the need to "ensure that the [family planning] services are of adequate quality and culturally acceptable"[23] indicated that, in 1972, from the birth controllers' point of view, all was not well. In 2001, a Labour government would spend £60million on schemes aimed at reducing teenage pregnancies (though without acknowledging that some of these teenagers, especially from ethnic minorities, might actually be married). Under this scheme, girls as young as 12 can obtain abortifacient morning-after pills, and paid 'pregnancy co-ordinators' are to counsel pregnant schoolgirls, accompanying them to the abortion clinic if necessary.[24]

Birth control advocates like Susan Hampshire, who on visiting the slums of Chittagong for the first time, and being "hit by the heat and the over-powering smell from the open drains...mingling with strange cooking smells", have pondered on why people who (they believe) need it most, do not practice birth control: "It would be wonderful if all the people who are physically capable of having children were educated on the facts of parenthood, to help them decide whether or not they really want them." She added: "Having more children than you can care for is madness".[25]

Hampshire must have been reassured by her encounter with a poor woman, lying on the floor of her hut, "[with] her 8 children – all covered in weeping sores due to malnutrition. The mother said faintly 'Now I accept family planning'. Despite her weak condition she smiled."[26]

Kingsley Davis says of the 'problem woman': "Her attitude is construed as due to ignorance and 'cultural values', and the policy deemed necessary to change it is 'education'. No compulsion can be used, because the movement is committed to free choice, but movie strips, posters, comic books, public lectures, interviews, and discussions are in order. These supply information and supposedly change values by discounting superstitions and showing that unrestrained procreation is harmful to both mother and children. The effort is considered successful when the woman decides she wants only a certain number of children and uses an effective contraceptive."[27]

Like the early birth controllers, who offered sewing classes with their homely birth control talks, modern population control charities promote the use of 'integrated' programmes, whereby birth control is offered in conjunction with other services. But what if the other services are taken up, while birth control is rejected?

Finding the Right Method

Birth controllers are fortunate in being able to study what amounts to an enormous long-running experiment in fertility limitation in the industrialised nations to discover what will work in poorer countries. Since it has been realised from the very beginning that contraception is fallible, birth controllers have had to acknowledge that a complete range of fertility control measures is needed to stop the poor having children. As in the BCC Report of 1972, these include sterilisation, abortion, and any new long-term birth control methods.[28] Despite the admission that abortion is necessary because of contraceptive failure, funds are still requested for contraception in order to prevent abortion.[29]

Each method has its pros and cons – but not necessarily the same pros and cons that the public might imagine. For example, when Elizabeth Draper discusses the American Food and Drug Agency medical survey on the IUD (from 8,000 questionnaires sent to Fellows of the American College of Obstetricians and Gynaecologists, eight deaths were found to be associated with the device, with 500 cases of severe illness), she says: "The major problems were infection and perforation of the uterus. Pain and increased bleeding were the most troublesome side effects. The latter made it unsuitable for couples forbidden intercourse during menstruation."[30]

Draper appears oblivious to the fact that a woman with severe bleeding would not wish, or even be able to, have intercourse, forbidden or otherwise. However, Draper is sensitive to the effect on prospective users of the serious health dangers posed by the IUD: "...a method which gets a bad name with the individual is not in the long term a good population controller...and risks discrediting other methods too".[31] The main worry about the bad side effects of contraceptives appears to be that they will put off women from using them.

What tends to happen in practice is that in the "long term", when a method such as the IUD is thoroughly discredited, a new 'safer' device will rise up to take its place. Meanwhile, Draper admits: "The device has been widely used in developing countries, inserted by medical and paradmedical personnel, some working in mobile treatment units". She adds: "Its failure rate and complications are probably higher than estimated as patients do not always return to the original clinic or doctor to report".[32] If it was inserted in a mobile treatment unit, it might be *impossible* for a woman to return and request the removal of the device, as Draper herself realises: "...disasters have occurred when no medical aid was within reach for removal".[33]

Turning from the study of past contraceptive disasters, to a disaster yet-to-come, Draper describes a "small device with copper like a finned flat-fish, called the Dalkon Shield, [which] has been found in trial to be nearly as effective as oral contraception. But researchers warn that trials tend to be more successful than subsequent general use, and there are pharmacological hazards".[34]

While realising that routine abortion as a method of birth control is not a practical option - it would be costly to provide, and women would be damaged by its frequent use – birth controllers have recognised that it is nevertheless essential because contraception frequently fails,[35] especially among young women and girls, who are more fertile.

Sterilisation is considered preferable – not because it does not destroy foetal life, as in abortion, but because an abortion can stop only one baby, while sterilisation is permanent. Indeed, Halliday Sutherland pointed out in 1936 that despite the relaxation of the Ministerial ban on contraceptive advice there had been "...no appreciable reduction in the large families of the poor..." and in view of this, the "failure of contraceptives as a means of social amelioration has been followed by a demand for sterilisation."[36]

However, because sterilisation is permanent, people are inclined to think more carefully about it. While female sterilisation can be reversed, the male procedure is more difficult, and anyway the male method is more efficient. (It is commoner for women to conceive after sterilisation.) Draper admits: "... medical facilities for mass treatment for reversal (re-anastomosis) do not exist in countries like India so that for all practical purposes there it must still be regarded as permanent, though the possibility of easy reversal would greatly facilitate acceptance in some cases."[37] In other words, if a permanent method of birth control were *not* permanent, people might want it!

In poor countries, reversal of sterilisation is no easy matter. Countries where – as the campaigners acknowledge - there are few health services, sterilisation reversal operations are unlikely to be offered as a priority to the poor. In any case, a country sufficiently committed to population control to permit widespread sterilisation, is unlikely to jeopardise such programmes by offering easy access to reversal operations.

In *Food, Saris and Sterilization: Population Control in* ,[38] Betsy Hartmann and Hilary Standing describe how women in were given food relief on condition that they were sterilised. The operations frequently left women weak (with "cut stomachs") and unable to work. Indira Gandhi, when Prime Minister of India, stirred enormous controversy with her coercive programmes of sterilisation during the 1970s. At first, Mrs Gandhi was opposed to coercion, but others were not so squeamish.

The US Agency for International Development (USAID), and the World Bank, with the help of some of India's elite, over-stepped the 'voluntary' mark, and 'family planning' became population control. When, in 1975, the Indian

Supreme Court declared Mrs Gandhi's election invalid, she declared a State of Emergency, suspending all civil liberties. By the end of the Emergency, in 1977, 6.5 million men had been sterilised, many by force.[39] 1,774 people died as a direct result of the operation. Robert Whelan remarks: "Western population lobbyists were delighted, not embarrassed, by the Indian government's performance".[40]

And what of the 'poor women'? Germaine Greer comments: "Two thousand rupees[41] is two hundred days' wages for a tea-plucker, but who wants the gold, she or her husband? Who dies in the yearly visitations of infectious disease guaranteed by the polluted water-supply and primitive hygiene in the estate-workers' village? Why, the babies of course. For the planters, two thousand rupees is an investment in continued productivity from the female worker and reduced health and educational expenses, but for her? Her sons might have rescued her from picking two-leaves-and-a-bud, two-leaves-and-a-bud for the rest of her life. What happens to a sterilised wife whose babies die? Her husband casts her off".[42]

But, like many another country subjected to population control, was not poor. A US Senate study found that it was "rich enough in fertile land, water, manpower and natural gas for fertiliser not only to be self sufficient in food, but a food exporter, even with rapidly increasingly population size". Despite (or perhaps because of) this, the World Bank, USAID and their allies in the Government enthusiastically espoused the programme.[43]

The perfect family planning method for most people is one that is likely to be safe, instant, reversible, does not interfere with enjoyment, and does not impinge on human dignity. In other words, fertility that can be turned on and off like a tap.

However, the population controller's ideal 'family planning' is something that is as long-lasting as possible, cannot be reversed by the client, and whose possible side effects can be quietly tried on those unable to complain, or sue, if anything goes wrong, and whose minor effects can be blamed on the recipient. Poor people – preferably living in poor countries, with little chance of stirring publicity - are ideal for the purpose.

Some early birth controllers, like Gladys Cox, puzzled as to the cause of side effects of contraceptives which were not suffered by all users, fell back on consigning responsibility for these side effects to individuals she evidently regarded as troublesome, as she confided in personal correspondence: "...I can only conclude that some patients are hypersensitive to all forms of chemical contraceptives. At Walworth yesterday, a patient told me that she experienced severe vaginal discomfort – 'a feeling as if boiling water were running through her vagina' – for several hours after using Volpar paste and soluble. The only chemical contraceptive which so far I have not known to cause irritation and discomfort is Milsan. The majority use chemicals without any discomfort; a small minority complain of irritation and 'stinging' from using the same chemical".[44]

The story of Margaret Sanger's and Gregory Pincus' experiments with the contraceptive pill in Puerto Rico is told in *Sex and Destiny*: "Like Stopes and Sanger…and all the birth controllers in history, Pincus was convinced that the poor were multiplying too fast. On America's doorstep there was a whole colony of C3 parents, in Stopesian terminology: Puerto Rico".[45] Linda Grant relates how threats and warnings were used against female medical personnel reluctant to be used as 'guinea pigs', because impoverished Peurto Rican women - allegedly crying out for birth control - did not rush to try out the Pill.[46]

In their report on the injectable method of birth control Depo-Provera, the women's campaign against the drug draws attention to a similar enthusiasm for experimentation. In view of its dangers,[47] campaigners argued that Depo-Provera should not be used on women anywhere. They plead: "What are the options for a woman who is poor, lives in the Third World and comes to the decision that she wants contraception? Increasingly, the only form of contraception available to her is likely to be a hormonal method or an IUD. It is eagerly provided by the clinic, without adequate checks or follow-up because she is no more than another statistic representing 'X' number of births prevented".

What was the response to this campaign? "On the whole, the women's movement in Europe and North America has not asked what lies behind the fact that women in Third World countries are often inundated with propaganda and inducements not to have babies".[48]

Similar controversy has dogged the use of the long-term Norplant®, an implanted hormonal device, which has been used on women in both poor and rich countries, often with disastrous results. Developed by the US-based Population Council, it was used in 'pre-introductory trials' in Brazil in 1984.[49] The implants caused menstrual chaos. The rods were supposed to have been left in place for not more than five years, but in some cases, when the women went to have them removed, the doctor in question was nowhere to be found. Some still had the implants in their arms six and a half years after research had begun. The women participating in the trial were poor, from the *favelas* of. After the trial was discontinued – under political pressure - they were still poor. They were also sick.

For many years, vast amounts of money have been poured into the incredibly dangerous pregnancy vaccination programme. Massive research is currently being supported by the World Health Organisation, an arm of the United Nations.[50] Pregnancy vaccination has long held a fascination for birth controllers.[51] It ties in with the philosophy that pregnancy is a disease that should receive priority treatment, and funds from health service budgets. The vaccination works by interfering with the body's natural tendency to recognise that, although the fertilised egg is genetically different from the mother, her immune system will not attack it as it would infectious micro-organisms, such as viruses, bacteria, parasites, or fungi.

Normally, the foetus's developing immune system also treats maternal cells, though genetically different, as self-like. Immune contraceptives work by interfering with maturation of eggs and production of sperm. They also interfere with fertilisation, implantation and development of early embryos – in other words, as an abortifacient.[52] The dangers posed by a preparation which interferes with the body's immune systems are immense – particularly in the light of experience regarding HIV and AIDs.

Richter, an opponent of dangerous methods, highlights the birth controllers' priorities in the search for the 'perfect' contraceptive: "A major driving force behind contraceptive development since the 1960s has been the aim to limit population growth. New contraceptives are designed to be highly effective, long lasting and independent of the user's whims or abilities. To effectively reduce birth rates, it is assumed that there should be no failures due to improper use or 'forgetting to take a pill'. Whether or not a woman can stop using a contraceptive any time she wishes has been less of a priority."[53]

Such drugs are recommended for the use of poor women because they lack access to health services, but without health services, there will be no proper monitoring of their use, and possible side effects will not be fully investigated. If the birth control method relies on a health professional for its removal, and the health professional vanishes, then any talk of 'choice' for women is empty rhetoric. It is precisely because the poor have so little choice in their lives that they are tempted to 'choose' the only thing that is offered.

Birth control, seen as beneficial or neutral in developed countries, can be used as a weapon. In countries under military occupation, long-term sterilising methods can be used against the conquered populace as just another method of repression. In East Timor, women complained that the Indonesian forces which illegally occupied their island in 1975, were trying to reduce their numbers by secretly injecting them with contraceptives under the guise of immunisations.[54]

The arms industries of Western nations had invested heavily in Indonesia.[55] The consequent lack of Western interest in their plight may have stemmed from the fact that contraception is seen as acceptable and desirable in the West. How could it possibly be used as a weapon? The Indonesian occupying forces pursued a policy of introducing its own settlers to the island, while dealing harshly with the native population.

Obviously birth control can be used as a weapon against one's enemies, just as easily, but not so visibly, as guns and tanks.[56] Often a harvest of resentment is reaped by rich countries which are seen as oppressors because of population control programmes. Ironically, such programmes are not the result of democratic debate or the popular will of people in the richer countries, who are just as surely targeted by population control. As George Grant points out, when in 1967 Tito invited Planned Parenthood to help "target certain sectors of [Yugoslav] society…" especially "troublesome concentrations of Croats and Slovenes, the scattered Moslem, Catholic, Lutheran, and Bohemian Reformed communities in Bosnia, Kosovo, and Dalmatia…" he attracted little attention.

107

However, when guns and concentration camps were employed against these culturally diverse communities, it was called ethnic cleansing, and the world intervened.[57]

The abortion drug RU486, previously banned in the United States because of safety fears, was given out free in New York clinics in trials conducted by Abortion Rights Mobilisation (ARM) in a bid to win the approval of the US Food and Drug Administration.[58]

Persuasion or Coercion?

There is an element of coercion here that will not have escaped those concerned with human rights. Because what people want to do, and what they are constrained to do by economic and social pressures, are two very different things. When people are poor, with very little real power over their lives, they may accept things that no rich, socially empowered person would accept without a fight. Those in positions of power can easily persuade themselves that they know what other people need.

A social worker who has written about birth control in the community, Elphis Christopher, illustrates the ease with which persuasion can become compulsion when the balance of social power is tilted: "When a woman (or couple) is reluctant or refuses to use contraception even though it would be in her own or her family's best interests the social worker will need to decide what to do about this."[59] Simply transpose the words "woman" and "social worker" to see the point. Familiar as we are with compulsory birth control in a country like China, we tend to overlook the more subtle pressures exerted in a democracy.

While stressing that compulsion is out of the question, birth control advocates have a habit of leaving the threat hanging in the air. Kingsley Davis drew attention to the social reformers who are normally happy with schemes such as compulsory unionisation, but who "balk at any suggestion that couples be permitted to have only a certain number of offspring.... Put the word *compulsory* in front of any term describing a means of limiting births – *compulsory sterilization, compulsory abortion, compulsory contraception* – and you guarantee violent opposition." He concludes: "Fortunately, such direct controls need not be invoked..."[60]

Similarly, George Morris canvassed several extreme measures of population control, but rejected them on the plea that "most of them" would be "morally unacceptable" or would infringe liberty or inflict hardship. As always, there are obstacles to consider, not least the democratic system: "Given the present state of public opinion, there would be no chance of these methods being introduced in any democracy". He concludes, somewhat wistfully: "Almost all the suggested methods would seem to be administratively unworkable". However, he goes on to warn that "if we do not act quickly in more conventional ways our children may have to resort to many of these methods." Morris's list of "unacceptable methods", to which he obviously gave careful thought, were:

1. No family allowances after the third or subsequent children.

2. Limitation of medical treatment, maternity benefits, housing and free schooling for families with more than a certain number of children.

3. Mass use of sterilants in the water supplies and food.

4. Two-tier marriage systems with only one group being eligible to produce children.

5. Licences to have children.

6. Temporary sterilisation of girls and women after childbirth.

7. Compulsory sterilisation for men with three or more living children.

8. Wealthy nations such as the United States insisting on population control as the price of food and other aid to developing countries.

9. Euthanasia.

10. Infanticide.[61]

Many of these bear an uncanny resemblance to population control measures employed in China where there is no democracy, and there is indeed a "massive system of informers and agents to ensure that…compulsory sterilization and abortion [take] place."[62]

Morris wrote his book, in which he apparently rejects extreme measures, in 1973. By 1976, he was arguing for fertility control units to be set up within the NHS – run on the lines of the 'charity organisations', which would provide contraception, abortion and sterilisation. These were necessary because, he claimed, Britain's population needed to be reduced to about 33million – between two-thirds and half what it then was.[63] It is difficult to understand how this was to have been accomplished without some of the drastic measures he had previously rejected.

Family planning surveys have repeatedly shown that, under ideal circumstances, people would like *more*, not *less*, children. Poor people, with less in the way of material distractions, actually welcome children for their freshness, absolute loyalty, unconditional love, and unpredictable capacity to amuse. They delight in their closeness and companionship in a way that would baffle many in economically developed societies.

At the height of the population explosion scare, opinion polls revealed a variety of conflicting views held by those members of the public questioned. While 45% thought that two children constituted the ideal family size, only 2% thought *no* children best, while 2% thought six or more! 83% approved of married couples using contraception to delay starting a family, but 62% thought large families should not be condemned. The opinions were not influenced by religion, since 60% questioned said the Church should "keep out of political matters". This seems to indicate a high level of public support for individuals choosing for themselves. However, since the majority of people questioned (52%) placed "economic affairs" at the top of their list of most urgent problems (population was not mentioned – only 10% named "international affairs" as their priority), it is likely that few members of the public were actually losing sleep over the population question.[64]

Given this indication of public indifference to population problems –
especially their opposition to criticism of large families – population
campaigners Potts and Selman continued to muse on those who "… have
argued that family planning programmes should be replaced by genuine
'population control' policies, which would concentrate on countering ingrained
desires to have large numbers of children."[65] These would operate by "educating
people into wanting fewer children, by attempting to change institutions which
support high fertility and by providing disincentives to having many children".
Far from reflecting public opinion, they sought to shape it to their own ends.

They pointed to Kingsley Davis, who saw 'family planning' as a distraction
from the real issues involved – not a distraction from poverty and inequality,
but from the need to reduce births. The key to the dedicated birth controller is,
apparently, not to make circumstances ideal - because in ideal circumstances
people would have more children - but to make circumstances harder.

In 1969, at the IPPF Conference in Dacca, Bernard Berelson, then
President of the Population Council, listed possible strategies in *Beyond Family
Planning*, which included the addition of sterilants to water/food supplies,
licences to have children, compulsory sterilisation of men with three or more
living children, abortion of all illegitimate pregnancies, financial incentives for
contraception and sterilisation and withdrawal of benefits and health care for
those with over a certain number of children and encouragement of women to
join the workforce to reduce fertility. 'Abortion camps' were a possibility for
developing countries and "compulsory methods would probably be quite
effective in lowering fertility".[66]

Absorbed as they are in the issue of population control, it is perhaps
understandable that some birth control advocates lose patience with those who
– as they see it – are determined not to be helped, as does A.S. Parkes: "It is
sometimes said that the development of the perfect contraceptive method
would solve the population problem. This I do not believe. For one thing, there
will never be a method perfect for use at all times, under all conditions, in all
parts of the world, and in all cultures. For another, the best of methods will be
of no value if it is not used, and here we have to face the problem of
motivation."

Getting to the root of the problem, he goes on: "Parental and especially
maternal urge is strong; even now there are wives who are not happy unless they
have young babies to look after."[67]

Coercion has been a feature of the birth control campaign since the
beginning. In 1877, Annie Besant, as we have seen, wanted society to
disapprove of large families.[68] Bessie Drysdale, writing in 1925, declared: "By
one means or another – example, instruction, compulsion even if necessary –
the stream of unwanted children must be stopped."[69] Janet Chance also
approved of compulsory birth control.[70] Both Stopes and Sanger supported
coercive sterilisation of the unfit.[71]

In so doing, they were following in the footsteps of Aristotle and Plato. Aristotle advocated birth control to achieve a stable population and avoid poverty. He also recommended abortion for any woman over 40, women who had borne the allotted number of children and infanticide for 'deformed' infants.[72] Plato suggested that reproduction be legally regulated. He approved of abortion for population control and recommended infanticide for eugenic reasons.[73] Both philosophers are treated unjudgementally by birth control historians.

Aristotle and Plato would feel at home in modern China, where coercion is used in the most blatant way to force women to contracept, abort or be sterilised. Husbands, families, neighbours and work-mates are also penalised.[74] Despite human rights protests, Western governments seem keener to make money out of the Chinese people by their production of cheap goods, than to protest their reproductive rights.[75]

Far from being shunned by the family planners, China has been praised.[76] Perhaps, also, China is useful as a warning – something campaigners are fond of – to keep the rest of the poor world in line. Nafis Sadik, head of the UNFPA, suggests (despite the Cairo Conference pledge to eliminate "all kinds of violence against women"):[77] "China could offer its experiences and special experts to other countries".[78] The message from Draper et al, veiled in liberal language, is that the poor must use birth control voluntarily, or they will be forced to do it.[79]

However horrific the methods used, nothing is so bad as not using them. Delia Davin, noting the "human cost" of the one-child family policy in China, the "horror of female infanticide" and that "[M]illions of women [have been forced] to undergo abortions which they would prefer not to have", nevertheless concludes: "Against all these must be balanced the potential cost of inaction".[80]

Even while explicitly rejecting the *idea* of coercion, family planners unconsciously use the *language* of coercion, and nobody seems to notice, or even care very much – especially when the verbal bullying is directed at those with little chance of answering back. Thus Baroness Chalker, former Secretary of State for Overseas Development, while boasting of the family planning schemes supported by the Overseas Development Administration ("None uses coercion"), proclaims in the title of her article: "Children *must not* be a matter of chance." [My italics][81] She goes on: "Poor countries *must* acknowledge...that population control is in their own interests."[82] [My italics]

Her contradictory sentiments are repeated in a kind of mantra that soothes liberal conscience on the population issue, expressed succinctly in a letter to the left-wing press: "Yes, social justice is a prerequisite for population control, but another essential is that having more than two children becomes socially unacceptable, everywhere."[83]

The theme of social and peer pressure to control population, expounded by Besant, is snatched up today by those with an interest in 'family planning', as in these sentiments expressed by the Secretary-General of the IPPF: "It [family planning] must mean taking the interests of all the family – and possibly the wider interests of the community and the country – into account when deciding to have a child..."[84]

A.S. Parkes states bluntly: "The Universal Declaration of Human Rights, issued by the United Nations in 1968, states that men and women have a right to marry and found a family, but ignores the question of family size. ...I would give a high place to an obligation not to produce children in demographically excessive numbers..."[85]

A kind of 'good cop/bad cop' scenario is played out, with official population bodies speaking softly, and eminent individuals conspicuously *outside* the population control machine, waving a big stick. For example, Professor Sir Roy Calne, world-renowned transplant surgeon, and father of six, proposed that couples should apply for a licence to have children, and that there should be a tax penalty for parents with more than two. He also suggested that it might be possible to create a virus as a fertility limiter.

Though denying charges of coercion, he suggested a population control laboratory situated in Delhi, Manila, Cairo or Rio, "somewhere...those coming to work each day would be reminded of the problems."[86] Like Bradlaugh before him, Calne clearly sees people as problems, and prophesied about mass migration and conflict, if governments failed to act. As before, population control was laid before us as a lesser evil – the greater evil being, of course, people.

The Secretary-General of the IPPF has expounded this theme of people-as-threat: "Adolescents represent a large and increasing sector of the population. By the year 2000 there will be little over one billion of them."[87]

There are still some people who persist in seeing poverty, not people, as the problem. They have more detailed knowledge of poverty than anyone, excepting the poor themselves: the charities who work with the poor, who have stubbornly refused to swallow the overpopulation theory of the causes of world poverty. However, pressure could be applied to make them change their minds. In 1994, the All-Party Parliamentary Group on Population and Development called for a doubling of government aid for population control, and a cut in aid to organisations that do not promote family planning.[88] More recently, one MP has been excluded from a Parliamentary committee concerned with international development on the grounds that he might be opposed to abortion and contraception,[89] and it has been suggested that the present Pope has been less of a "force for good" in the developing world than in eastern Europe, because he is "so opposed to birth control".[90]

Abstinence – Makes the Heart Grow Fonder?

With all the problems and dangers of birth control, surely abstinence (the best method of birth control, if we view it in such a narrow way) deserves a higher profile? Yet birth controllers, from Annie Besant and the Drysdales, have felt the need to warn against it. Some used truly alarming threats, as did nineteenth century physician, T. A. McGraw, who claimed: "[A]bstention when the prevention of conception was indicated would only drive the husband to the brothel."[91] George Drysdale actually believed that prostitution was caused by celibate women, because they 'forced' men to seek out prostitutes.[92]

It was Malthus, scorned for his rejection of contraception, who at least realised that abstinence was the only sure way to prevent births. Yet as recently as 1994, the FPA sponsored a visit by SIECUS (the Sex Information & Education Council of the United States) to warn the UK against the abstinence programmes for young teens which have been gaining in popularity in the United States.[93] Their fears might have been justified if the programmes had been shown to be defective – but evidence shows that they have been a resounding success, not just in preventing teenage births, but in raising youngsters' self-esteem.[94]

Nevertheless, abstinence appears to be regarded as a threat by birth controllers. Recently a massive donation was made to the UN by Ted Turner, head of American media giant CNN and co-chairman of Time-Warner. Turner was reported to be keen to finance United Nations projects through his charitable foundation, the United Nations Foundation. The first $20million of a $1billion gift to the UN would be earmarked for special causes, such as population, women, environmental change and children's health.[95] At the same time Turner's then wife, actress Jane Fonda – also with an interest in population matters, and a UN 'goodwill ambassador'[96] - spear headed the campaign against abstinence.[97]

Perhaps the point about abstinence is that it leads people to think that they should not enter into a sexual relationship unless they wish to start a family, and that it may be wise to check whether their intended partner is of similar mind. It also draws attention to the fact that contraception sometimes fails. Perhaps – paradoxically - it concentrates the mind *too much* on reproduction. A birth controller's ideal contraceptive is one that *severs* the connection between sex and reproduction, which is why the Pill was such a breakthrough.[98] It is not necessary to be in a sexual relationship to take the Pill. Teenagers are prescribed it for any number of complaints, such as acne, period pains, or even absence of periods,[99] and the health pages of magazines and newspapers are littered with tales of medical problems caused or exacerbated by the indiscriminate prescription of artificial hormones. The idea has already been planted in the minds of young girls that a 'medicine' can be used for contraceptive purposes if they so choose.

Now that the threat of the brothel has receded, it has been replaced by the threat of teenage pregnancy. Whereas ailing wives were once warned that if they did not use contraception, their husbands would resort to prostitutes, parents are now warned that if they prevent their children from gaining access to contraception, they will be responsible for unwanted pregnancies. Young people are determined to have sex anyway, it is alleged; parents should ensure that they are at least 'prepared' with contraceptives, so that even eleven-year-olds have been recommended the pill. Parents are now being seen as an obstacle - preventing children obtaining contraception, as a recently issued training pack for GPs demonstrates. The pack includes suggestions for dealing with difficult situations faced by GPs when advising young people about contraception, such as "getting a parent out of the room".[100]

Despite talk of 'raging hormones', there is evidence that very young teenagers are much more socially conservative than the sex educators are suggesting.[101] However, explicit sex education material for youngsters helps break the link between sex and reproduction, because it encourages the young to engage in sex at an early age.[102] Most people would not associate 'family planning' with thirteen-year-olds. It is patently obvious that they cannot marry, live independently, or found a family. However, by aiming contraception specifically at the very young, the idea is implanted that sex is for fun, while reproduction is a serious matter, only to be undertaken by a mature adult.

With more young people engaging in sex, more conceptions are taking place, helped by greater fertility and less expertise with contraception, though even those who have sought contraceptive advice have quickly fallen pregnant.[103] However, it is not the increased *pregnancies* that are problematical for population controllers, but the fact that not all young girls are aborting.[104]

Despite the fact that only a minority of youngsters is affected by teenage pregnancy, it is seen as a matter of the utmost urgency to get *all* youngsters to contracept, and to steer them towards abortion when contraception fails. Family planners have expressed concern that some ethnic minority students and those attending religious schools may not be reached by sex education,[105] but the use of the internet has ensured that parental influence can now be by-passed.[106]

Cutting teenage pregnancies was made a priority by John Major's government, and the baton has been handed on smoothly to their Labour successors.[107] Governments of all political hues have continued to consult family planning organisations on this growing problem of modern society, but have failed to consult parents. They have given ever-more generous funding to contraceptive policies, despite glaring evidence that such policies do not work – in fact, that they appear to stimulate the very behaviour that most people wish the young to avoid.

Undeterred by manifest failure, the FPA in 1997 issued a leaflet entitled 'It doesn't matter how old you are', clearly aimed at young teenagers – or even younger children – with its bright colours, illustrations of make-up, purses, brightly-packaged sanitary towels, and opened condom packets. It shows a young person's bus pass, and a birthday cake, apparently decorated with twelve candles.[108] The leaflet also contains advice regarding 'morning-after contraception' (abortifacients), and contact numbers for organisations that refer youngsters for abortion.

The morning-after pill is now a central part of the present Government's drive against teenage pregnancy, despite admissions that the procedure has not been tested on young girls.[109] On questioning, the Department of Health denied that 'morning-after' pills act as abortifacients, stating that the "consensus of medical and legal advice" was that "pregnancy begins at implantation in the endometrium". With a marked lack of logic, they continue: "Post-coital intervention takes place before implantation" (it was not revealed how this could be known) "and is therefore a method of contraception and not abortion".[110] Meanwhile, the consensus of medical literature (obviously not the "advice" sought by, and given to, the Government) continues to regard conception as the beginning of life.

For some years, it has been suggested that celibacy is outmoded and unworkable. Agony Aunt Anna Raeburn, has stated flatly: "Sexual abstinence is possible but the assumption of its being carried out on a mass scale is not practical."[111] The fact that celibacy can be a positive lifestyle choice that is actually being lived out by many individuals, is therefore seen as a threat. Such examples of chastity explode the myth that a celibate lifestyle is impossible. Perhaps this explains Professor A.S. Parkes' attack on the "effrontery" of (unspecified) individuals, who "themselves practising the ultimate form of birth-control, attempt to ban more practical methods for other people."[112]

Magazines aimed at girls from twelve upwards (though even younger girls read them) have also come under fire for their concentration on value-free sex,[113] which again is coupled with contact numbers for abortion referral agencies, listed as 'advice' centres.[114] A Victorian feminist could be forgiven for thinking that such magazines were specially designed by unprincipled libertines whose aim was to debauch very young girls.

The articles are tawdry, and the answers to the pathetic 'problem' letters are cold and lacking in compassion, despite their jokey terminology. It is as though a brisk libertarian broom has been employed to sweep away the embarrassing wreckage of young lives caused by putting those libertarian theories into practice. Youngsters are told brusquely to get real, and stop whining about the negative outcomes of sexual encounters. Despite the fact that 'free sex' sounds like a great idea, it is clear that someone is paying the price.

Only after some high-profile criticism[115] have teenage magazines started to emphasise the age of consent on their problem pages which, however, continue to explain the physical aspects of a variety of sexual practices in cool, scientific language, no doubt in line with the philosophy of giving children factual information and leaving them to make up their own minds what to do with it. A panel has been formed to 'monitor' the magazines, but it is composed of magazine representatives.[116] However, the magazines have been used to advertise the Government-sponsored web site previously referred to, which children of any age can access.

This orchestrated alarm over under-age pregnancies should alert us to the possibility that this is merely a prelude to some sort of action overseas – however, more of that later. In the meantime, in Western countries drastic, and even ludicrous, measures have been used to deter young girls from becoming mothers. Some authorities employ a plastic baby doll that 'cries' until its 'needs' are met. It has been given to young school pupils in a bid to warn them that babies are not cute, cuddly things, but nasty, screaming, demanding little creatures. Conscientious pupils, who regularly see to the 'baby's needs', are awarded high marks.

What seems to have been overlooked, however, is the fact that such conscientious pupils will be the ones to hesitate over starting a family ("Tobi really put me off having kids," remarked one fourteen-year-old, given a 'B' for 'parenting skills'), while the pupil who ruthlessly chucks the doll in the dustbin in response to its 'crying' will probably go blithely ahead and have children.

The doll, designed by a NASA scientist, appears to replicate the negative aspects of child rearing, and thus neatly dovetails with the birth controllers' negative image of babies. Young working-class girls, though apparently fit to look after the children of others for a small wage, should not be entrusted with the care of their own.[117]

Reinforcing the notion that young girls need to be taught that, though sex is value-free, babies are bad, TV soap operas, aimed at a wide audience, have featured with monotonous regularity the theme of unplanned pregnancies being treated as a disaster worse than a terminal illness. This is an intriguing innovation for Western countries, as TV soap operas have been used in Third World countries for many years to teach the poor to limit their families.

However, since abortion is legal in most Western countries, it is now routinely introduced as an 'option' for pregnant TV characters. Abortion advocate Suzanne Moore, commenting on the sexual themes of a popular TV 'soap', enthused:

"Our acceptance of these storylines demonstrates, whatever politicians may say, that we are basically a liberal nation, that the moral sophistication required to navigate our way through these confusing times is indeed being learnt somehow. The evidence for this may well lie in the appeal of Eastenders and many other soaps to young people. They act as a primary source of sex education. No, they do not tell you exactly how to put on a condom, but they deal with the messiness of love, sex, the whole shebang, in a way that neither school nor parents can or will."[118]

The Government has not been slow in recognising the educative potential of popular drama, with health minister Yvette Cooper enthusing about under-age pregnancy story-lines due to appear on two rival TV 'soaps'.[119]

For generations, the birth controllers have faced the obstacle of women's reluctance to embrace their ideology, but television is a powerful medium, and cultural influences that encourage young girls to reject motherhood cannot be underestimated. 'Soaps' may not show a condom being used, but they can show that having a baby is not the inevitable outcome of having sex, when abortion is an option. Abortion and the morning-after pill can be used to mop up contraceptive disasters, if only the young can be taught to use them.

And contraceptive disasters continue to occur, despite (or perhaps because of) the calls of birth control organisations for ever-younger sex education. Rather than taking the opportunity these disasters afford to study the possible failures in their birth control programmes, proponents of contraception typically use any public concern about sexual activity in the young to call for even more sex education, and even more 'advice', at ever younger ages. So the family planning merry-go-round goes round, faster and faster. The casualties are the children, for whose welfare such schemes are supposed to be devised.[120]

Victoria Gillick, a long-time campaigner against prescribing contraception to minors without parental consent, is convinced that commercial interests in contraception depend on expanding the market for pills and condoms to young teenagers. She remarks: "No organisation with even the remotest connection with the provision, sale or trade in contraceptives should be allowed to dictate/advise sex education programmes, leaflets, reports, etc."

Though sexually active young teenagers are still in a minority, figures show staggering rises in provision of contraception and the morning-after pill. In 1994, 52,844 under-16s obtained contraceptives, rising to 89,315 in 1997. In only three years, from 1994 to 1997, the numbers of under-16s receiving 'morning-after treatment' rose from 8,604 to 23,060. In the four years from 1994 to 1998, under-age conceptions rose from 7,800 to 8,438.[121] Far from encouraging chastity for the very young, it would appear that there is a vested interest in encouraging sexual activity. Any profits made go to the drugs and contraceptive manufacturers, paid for by the tax-payer, while parents, who are no longer allowed to be informed when contraceptives are supplied to under-age girls, have to assume responsibility when things go wrong.[122]

Of less sensational interest than teenage pregnancies is the rising number of sexually transmitted diseases, one of the physical outcomes of youthful sexual activity.[123] One of the side effects of sexually transmitted diseases is that they can make women infertile. But if the proponents of contraception are less interested in female empowerment, and more interested in suppressing women's fertility for reasons of population control, they will not be too worried about that.

As a tragic postscript to this appalling saga of sexual abuse of the young in which successive governments have colluded, it has been reported that the number of men prosecuted for having sex with girls in recent years has slumped, despite evidence that the proportion of young girls engaging in sexual relations has risen dramatically.[124] It is a picture that would be familiar to the Victorians - with a couple of important differences. In Victorian times, no one in authority would have aided and abetted such abuse. Yet even if they had, they would have been roundly condemned by the feminist movement.

Back to Nature?

One method of family planning hitherto not discussed is Natural Family Planning. NFP is free, safe, reversible, does not impede pleasure or impair human dignity, and has no unpleasant, unhealthy or dangerous side effects. But – apart from the element of abstinence, which, as we have seen, is unacceptable to birth controllers – it is too closely tied to reproduction. For it can also be used to *have* children, by helping to pinpoint the time of ovulation, and also by keeping reproductive organs healthy by not subjecting them to the effects of powerful steroids. Because of this, it is not a perfect method of contraception for birth controllers, who continue to prophesy against it, stressing the difficulties involved. Despite this, scientific studies in various countries, rich and poor (including China) have revealed a high level of success with NFP.[125]

It is ironic that since the 'safe period' began to be really safe, it has not been recommended by birth controllers. In *Abortion*, Diggory, Potts and Peel suggest that using the 'safe period' increases the number of babies with abnormalities:

"A final poignancy is added by the fact that the one method of contraception recommended by Catholic thinkers may well be associated with an increase in some of the very abnormalities which abortion attempts to eliminate."[126] Thus they successfully implant a fear of natural methods by suggesting that the fertilisation of eggs at the end of the fertile period is responsible for larger numbers of congenital abnormalities, at the same time enjoying a joke at the expense of those foolish enough to reject both artificial contraception *and* abortion.

In case this interpretation should be thought too harsh, they also include a warning against the development of drugs to *prevent* miscarriage, because of the 'role' played by miscarriage in eliminating congenital abnormalities.[127] In other words, the misery of miscarriage must continue so that disabled babies may not be born. Their warning is repeated when assessing the relative risks to women of various fertility control methods (in which they include abortion).

The warning against the 'safe period' is echoed in a later work by Potts and Selman: "One small case-control retrospective study suggests a higher than usual incidence of congenital abnormality in children born to women using a rhythm method".[128] They go on to claim that the method, though not popular in any country (even Catholic countries) could be useful in "extending the pregnancy interval and, when linked with abortion, makes a powerful combination for fertility-control".[129] Here, the authors appear to damn the method, while simultaneously seeing the possibility of using its alleged inefficacy to encourage abortions. Perhaps it is a veiled encouragement to those women with objections to abortion, to use the pill instead.

Though the early Malthusians recommended the safe period (despite its unreliability), Norman Himes, in 1936, warns against it.[130] By this time, however, many important discoveries had been made regarding the process and timing of ovulation. In 1930, Ogino in Japan, and in 1931, Knaus in Austria, discovered by independent research that ovulation occurred twelve to sixteen days before the onset of menstruation.

Stopes' old adversary, Halliday Sutherland, who detailed the more accurate methods in *Laws of Life* (1936) and *Control of Life* (1947),[131] complete with perpetual calendars to take account of variations in cycles, has been largely ignored by birth control historians, apart from his role as protagonist in Stopes' libel action.[132] He is referred to as a 'Catholic doctor', with no mention of his interest in the 'safe period' - not even to condemn it.[133] Draper claims that the 'safe period' was tried in India, without success, but does not mention Sutherland.[134] Greer, though referring to Billings and Ogino-Knaus, does not mention Sutherland. Potts and Selman[135] fail to mention Sutherland, even to condemn him. Wood and Suitters mention Pouchet's findings regarding the female cycle, but only to praise him for his 'contraceptive' findings.[136]

Ruth Hall, in her biography of Marie Stopes, is more revealing, telling us that Sutherland had been on a whaling ship in Shetland, a doctor in Spain, and a naval surgeon during the War. He had done original work on tuberculosis and became deputy commissioner for TB medical services in England and Wales.[137] Perhaps the real reason for this neglect of Sutherland was because his arguments – though founded on religious ones - were political, containing more socialism and feminism than those of his opponents put together.

In characteristic style, Sutherland sets out to describe Malthusian claims and methods: "According to Malthusian doctrine overpopulation is the cause of poverty, disease and war: and consequently, unless the growth of population is artificially restrained, all attempts to remedy social evils are futile. Malthusians claim that 'if only the devastating torrent of children could be arrested for a few years, it would bring untold relief'. They hold that overpopulation is the root of all social evil, and the truth or falsehood of that proposition is therefore the basis of all their teaching. Now, when Malthusians are asked to prove that this their basic proposition is true, they adopt one of two methods, not of proof, but of evasion. Their first method of evading the question is by asserting that the truth of their proposition is self-evident and needs no proof. To that we can reply that the falsity of the proposition can and will be proved. Their second device is to put up a barrage of facts which merely show that all countries, and indeed the earth itself, would have been overpopulated long ago if the increase of population had not been limited by certain factors, ranging from celibacy and late marriages to famines, diseases, wars and infanticide."

He agrees these facts are "indisputable", but goes on to argue that it is a "manifest breach of logic" to claim, because poverty, disease, and war have checked an increase of population, that poverty, disease, and war are actually *caused* by an increase of population.[138]

Having attacked the basis of Malthusianism – that people are the cause of poverty – he goes on to lay bare the political and economic interests behind the Malthusian cause: "The Wages Fund Theory is an economic reflection of the Malthusian myth. This theory assumes that a definite fixed sum is available every year for distribution as wages amongst labourers, so that the more numerous the labourers the less wages will each one receive. From this theory the Malthusians argue that the only remedy for low wages is artificial birth control. They carefully refrain from telling the working classes the other aspect of this…theory – namely, that if the workers in one trade receive a rise in wages, a corresponding reduction must be made in the wages of others, so that a rise in wages here and there confers no real benefit on the labouring classes as a whole. That is merely one illustration of capitalist bias in the Malthusian propaganda. In any case, economic science has discarded the Wages Fund Theory as a pure fiction. No fixed or definite sum is available for wages, because the wages of a labourer are derived from the produce of his work."[139]

Sutherland argued that poverty was the cause, not the result, of a high birth rate. He maintains that Malthusian doctrine is a "barrier to social reform, because it implies that humane legislation, by encouraging population, will of necessity defeat the aim of those who desire to improve the conditions of the poor by methods other than the practice of artificial birth control".[140]

Under the blunt heading "Malthusianism is an Attack on the Poor", Sutherland continues: "Both the supporters and the opponents of Malthus are often mistaken in considering his greatest achievement to be a policy of birth control. Malthus did a greater and a more evil thing. He forged a law of nature, namely, that there is always a limited and insufficient supply of the necessities of life in the world. From this false law he argued that, as population increases too rapidly, the new-comers cannot hope to find a sufficiency of good things; that the poverty of the masses is not due to conditions created by man, but to a natural law; and that consequently this law cannot be altered by any change in political institutions. This new doctrine was eagerly adopted by the rich, who were thus enabled to argue that Nature intended that the masses should find no room at her feast; and that therefore our system of industrial capitalism was in harmony with the Will of God. Most comforting dogma!"

Sutherland delineates the process of acceptance, by the rich and powerful, in varying degrees, of Malthusian doctrine: "Without discussion, without investigation, and without proof, our professors, politicians, leader-writers, and even our well-meaning socialists, have accepted as true the bare falsehood that there is always an insufficient supply of the necessities of life; and today this heresy permeates all our practical politics. In giving this forged law of nature to the rich, Malthus robbed the poor of hope. Such was his crime against humanity. In the words of Thorold Rogers, Malthusianism was part and parcel of 'a conspiracy, conceived by the law and carried out by parties interested in its success, to cheat the English workman of his wages, to tie him to the soil, to deprive him of hope, and to degrade him into immediate poverty.'"

His concluding words must have worried Marie Stopes, who was to sue him for libel: "When Malthusians enter a slum for the purpose of preaching birth control, it is right that the people should be told what is written on the passports of these strangers."[141]

Meanwhile, Malthusians were uttering such compassionate statements as: "We must no longer be content to remain indifferent and idle witnesses of the senseless and unthinking procreating of countless wretched children, whose parents are diseased and vicious".[142] Sutherland agrees that "disease, vice, and wretched children are the saddest products of our industrial system", but maintains: "it is also true that a helpless baby never yet was guilty of expropriating land, of building slums, of under-paying the workers, or of rigging the market. Therefore instead of preventing the birth of children we should set about to rectify the evil conditions which make the lives of children and adults unhappy. Like many other policies advocated on behalf of the poor, birth control is immoral if only on this account, that *it distracts attention from the real causes of poverty*."[143] (My italics) He concludes by quoting Cardinal Manning, friend of the Trade Unions and the poor:

"There is a natural and divine law, anterior and superior to all human and civil law, by which men have the right to live of the fruits of the soil on which they are born, and in which they are buried."[144]

Another physician who argued against birth control was Dr Laetitia Fairfield. She receives even less mention in birth control histories than does Sutherland. Leathard refers to her thus: "In 1926, at the suggestion of Dr Halliday Sutherland and Dr Laetitia Fairfield, two Catholics who regarded birth control as a national peril, the League of National Life was formed to combat the theory and practice of birth prevention".[145] She goes on to say: "Opponents contended that birth control would eliminate the fitter stocks, put the British empire in jeopardy and lead to increased lunacy in women. It poisoned married life, degraded wives to mere gratifiers of lust and depraved unmarried women." The juxtaposition of Sutherland, Fairfield, and the League of National Life with such sentiments, suggests that these may have been their views. However, when we turn to the source of the latter remark, purporting to sum up the arguments of birth control opponents, we find that Leathard is in fact quoting an opinion expressed by Peter Fryer, in *The Birth Controllers*!

Fryer's own references to Fairfield are confined to her "elegant expression 'mutilated intercourse'," which she used to "describe the use of contraceptives"[146] and: "In 1926, Dr Halliday Sutherland suggested to his friend Dr Letitia (sic) Fairfield that an organization be formed to combat the theory and practice of birth control, which they both regarded as a national peril."[147]

To read Dr Fairfield's arguments, it is necessary to turn to the *Encyclopaedia of the Labour Movement Vol.I*. Her opening remarks are surprisingly down-to-earth, given the picture we now have of a slightly mad, narrow-minded, religious fanatic: "The arguments against birth control are difficult to present in small compass, because of the very wide issues involved, religious, medical, economic, and social. In the present controversy the term 'birth control' really means 'conception control by artificial means'." She goes on to allow for the fact that births may be restricted within marriage, for health reasons, or "apprehension for the welfare of the coming child, economic stress, etc."

121

Like Sutherland (she lists two of his books on birth control for further reading, so presumably drew on them for her contribution, but she also made a significant contribution to the campaign against sterilisation), she condemns Malthusian theory as false, saying that poverty in a family or community may be due to many forms of "bad distribution of wealth". As to medical reasons for using contraceptives, although pregnancy may have needed to be postponed for health reasons, she states: "...permanent or very prolonged prohibitions against child-bearing on strictly medical grounds are much rarer than is supposed."

She goes on to point out something that should have been self-evident to socialists: "Medical contra-indications to pregnancy tend to diminish as medical skill expands. In the hard cases of excessive child-bearing often quoted, the woman usually needs medical treatment, or complete marital rest, or encouragement and comfort."

There was at this time no free antenatal care, no family allowances and no free medical or obstetric care. Fairfield's simple arguments highlight a glaring omission in the demands of the birth control advocates. Far from making birth control opponents sound mad, it calls into question the good sense of some of its advocates.

Her allegations of the health effects of contraceptives ("sterility...local congestion...inflammation and sepsis...the tendency to tumour formation....serious nervous strain") do not sound so strange when one considers the substances which were used, the experiments which were made, and the motivations (certainly not women's health) that drove the birth control advocates.

Even worse for the birth control lobby, Fairfield also exposes the class arguments of socialist birth control advocates as hollow and callous. She continues to rub salt in a good many 'socialist' wounds: "The group of economist birth controllers before mentioned" [Dr Drysdale, President of the Neo-Malthusian League; Harold Cox; Major Leonard Darwin] "have issued the clearest warnings that birth control is to be regarded as a cheap alternative to social reform. If the State provides the working man with the means of limiting his family, money need no longer be squandered on rebuilding slums, on State education, etc. He will have children at his peril."

She quotes Drysdale: "Those who are relatively poor (which must be admitted to be evidence of economic unfitness) should only have the number of children they can rear without State or other aid."[148] This must have been a grave embarrassment to socialists like Dora Russell, because they worked alongside 'friends of the economically unfit' like Drysdale.

Russell, who gives the case *for* birth control in this volume, actually goes so far as to defend Malthusianism, including "Malthusian Arguments for Birth Control" in her contribution, which contains a great deal of information on the campaign for birth control in Parliament and the Labour Party. She claims: "The Neo-Malthusians...maintained that if people could be got to understand and to practice harmless artificial methods of family limitation, prosperity and comfort would speedily become far more widespread."[149]

Things are not always what they seem, and people do not always resemble their glowing portraits. The 'distinguished and eminent' have been lauded because they supported birth control, while opponents have been dismissed as "Catholic". Laetitia Fairfield, however, had credentials which some birth control advocates would have given their eye teeth for.[150] Significantly, she is also described in the *Encyclopaedia* as a member of the Executive of the Fabian Society (the socialist society), and Chairman of the Executive of the Church League for Woman's Suffrage. After the War, she was arguing within the Church for a comprehensive medical service.[151] The feminist Dora Russell is described as: "educated at Girton College, Cambridge", then details of her husband, the Hon. Bertrand Russell, are given: "Labour Candidate for Chelsea, 1924." Her publications are listed as: "Birth Control and the State" and "numerous articles".[152]

Fryer does mention Fairfield's post at the London County Council in *The Birth Controllers* (p247); but Leathard, in *The Fight for Family Planning*, unintentionally reveals a little more of Fairfield's credentials in an anecdote about the Second World War: "The FPA sought to make contraceptive advice available to married women in the forces through Army medical officers for whom the FPA would provide the teaching technique. Investigating Auxiliary Territorial Service provision, Dr Helena Wright discovered that their head of medical services was none other than the well-known opponent of birth control, Dr Letitia Fairfield."[153]

A Tangled Web

Sutherland's and Fairfield's arguments make their opponents' arguments look strange indeed, coming as they did from professed socialists and feminists. Sutherland's numerous works have been ignored. Even his embarrassing reference to the "coloured race" is not mentioned: "As things are, the original Protestant stock of America is being swamped by the growth of the Catholic, the Jewish, and the Negro population. Moreover, the United States is faced by the grave problem of a rapidly increasing coloured race."[154]

Taken on its own, this remark suggests – what? Certainly not that Sutherland advocated birth control for the "coloured race". He continues: "Despite this fact the American Malthusians are now demanding that a National Bureau should be established to disseminate information regarding contraceptives throughout their country!"[155] He uses this example as an attack on the ludicrousness of the Malthusians advocation of contraceptives which would not be used by the very people for whom they were intended (Catholics, Jews and blacks), among whom he himself is of course included.

It was Margaret Sanger and her allies among the rich and powerful who were keen to limit the fertility of blacks, Catholics and Jews, and the poor of all races, as were many British birth controllers. Sutherland did not rest his opposition to birth control on the idea of white hegemony, though he was concerned about the rise of population in Germany and Italy, against which he warned. (So were France, Belgium and Luxembourg, with memories of the First World War still fresh.)

He was an Imperialist, as were most British people of his time, and he argued against birth control partly because he believed that a thriving British population was essential in order to settle and administrate the British colonies. He did not, however, believe that birth control was a solution to poverty, and outlined economic solutions instead.

A true racist would have been selective in his application of birth control, but Sutherland was not. He believed artificial methods to be evil for anyone, whatever their origin, but was happy to support natural methods, providing they did not encroach on human dignity.

The reputation of a better-known anti-eugenicist, G.K. Chesterton, who argued brilliantly against the sterilisation campaign, has in recent years suffered from accusations of racism. Yet H.G. Wells, who not only supported forced sterilisation, but envisaged concentration camps for the 'unfit', has emerged with his reputation relatively unscathed.[156] Wells was pro-birth control, and Chesterton was not.

Stopes and Sanger, both of whom believed in forced birth control, have been gently handled by historians. Incredibly, it is Marie Stopes who is reported to have been 'disgusted' at Sutherland's attempts to "turn birth control into a political issue".[157] But birth control was already being used as a political instrument (what would nowadays be known as 'ethnic cleansing'), not least by Stopes herself. She, who could brook no opposition, was furious because someone had the temerity to challenge *her own* political use of birth control.

Stopes, who believed "Utopia could be reached in my lifetime had I the power to issue inviolable edicts"[158] also wanted legislation to compulsorily sterilise (among others) 'revolutionaries'. But she believed that by giving birth control to poor women, more revolutionaries could be prevented from coming into the world: "We have been breeding revolutionaries through the ages and at an increasing rate since the crowding into cities began…"[159] Both Stopes and Sanger were eugenicists, and Stopes' interest in eugenics certainly preceded her interest in birth control.[160]

Of Leathard's "impressive array" of thirty-four vice-presidents of the NBCC, "distinguished in the field of medicine, politics and sociology", those named - J. M. Keynes, Bertrand Russell, H.G. Wells, H.J. Laski, A.M. Carr-Saunders – were all involved in eugenics. So were the members of the Governing Body whom she mentions: Dr C.V. Drysdale, Ernest and Dorothy Thurtle and Dr C.P. Blacker. The members of the Executive Committee referred to as "similarly impressive" – Eva Hubback, Margery Spring-Rice, Mary Stocks, Marie Stopes and Dr Helena Wright – were all eugenicists.[161] This is by no means an exhaustive list. Indeed, it is hard to find a member of the original birth control campaign who was *not* involved in population control, or eugenics, or both.

The English Eugenics Society at first did not advocate contraception. They feared that, if widely adopted throughout society, it would be more likely to be used by the prudent individuals, those whom the eugenicists thought should be encouraged to have large families. They believed (correctly, as it turned out) that the poor would reject birth control.

Eugenicists were convinced that, as time went by, the poor would outbreed the wealthier sections of society, and at some point in the future would compose the majority of the population. At first, 'positive eugenics' (whereby those perceived by the Eugenics Society to be of superior stock were encouraged to marry and have large families) was espoused. There was animosity between eugenicists and Malthusians, because the Malthusians were against large families *per se*, while the eugenicists were keen for 'superior' people to have more children.

This animosity persisted, despite attempts by the Drysdales and other Malthusians to infiltrate the Eugenics Society and put the case for contraception. As was to be expected, the marriage was not a happy one, but after the First World War, a new wave of eugenically-minded women, including Stopes, championed birth control for the poor. Although they claimed to want birth control for egalitarian reasons, they hoped, via their clinics, to be able to encourage those whom they considered 'superior' or 'fit' to have *more* children.

Thus the case for birth control was finally won – not among the people, and certainly not among the poor, but among those who saw it as their business to control the reproduction of others.

Although the Malthusians were against *any* large families, they were eager to point out to the Eugenicists that they had always been keen on quality, as well as quantity, in the population. After all, was not their motto "*Non Quantitas, Sed Qualitas*"?[162] In 1922, C.V. Drysdale wrote a prophetic letter to the Eugenics Society:

"I feel quite sure that the neo Malthusian and Eugenic movements will come into ever closer relationship as times goes on…we of course can only represent one even though a very important side of the Eugenics question…before long we shall find the two movements agreed on all essential points, and it will always be our aim to direct birth control on the soundest eugenic principles. We shall be very glad of any co-operation you can give in securing this aim."[163]

This was part of a correspondence initiated by the Drysdales, in which the Eugenics Society appeared to distance itself from Neo-Malthusian ideas, while at the same time keeping the lines of communication open.[164]

The ideas of the two organisations were certainly in agreement on the subject of the working classes. C.V. Drysdale complained about the "large and irresponsible mass of people, who imagine that the State has an inexhaustible coffer from which they can get maternity bonuses, free education and feeding children, old age pensions, etc. merely by shouting loudly enough."[165]

Until the poor restricted their birthrate, he argued, "...the most truly democratic sociologist ought to have the gravest doubts as to the advisability of adult suffrage."[166] The birth control advocates - portrayed as champions of women's rights - would have accorded the poor no rights at all, had they the "power to issue inviolable edicts". What drove the Malthusians was fear of the poor, of what would happen if they ever issued forth from their slums and saw how people like Drysdale and Stopes lived.

Encouraged by irresponsible socialists, the poor were demanding ever greater benefits from the State, which would have to be paid out of the taxes of the rich. They were being given the vote, and through it, obtaining benefits - and all for 'nothing'. The Malthusians did not accept that the poor made any contribution to society at all, but saw them as so much useless lumber, cluttering up the otherwise tidy, prosperous world they inhabited.

NOTES

[1] See Jonathan Sacks, *The Politics of Hope*, Vintage, 2000, p.113.

[2] *Society and Fertility, op cit*, p208.

[3] For example, take-up of family allowances is practically 100%.

[4] *The Tamarisk Tree, op cit.*

[5] *The Fight for Family Planning, op cit.*

[6] *ibid*

[7] "There are those who are trapped, whether through ignorance or superstition, incapacity or instinct, by their habit of multiplying their numbers without limit." (C.D. Darlington, *The Little Universe of Man*, George Allen & Unwin, 1978, p269)

[8] "From my personal contact on Merseyside...large numbers of Catholics were desperately hoping for a less stringent attitude to the 'lesser evil'." [The contraceptive pill as against abortion] (Edwin Brooks, *This Crowded Kingdom*, p110)

[9] See *Society and Fertility, op cit.*

[10] *Feminism and Family Planning in Victorian England, op cit*, p130.

[11] *Population, Evolution and Birth Control, op cit*, p348.

[12] *Birth Control in the Modern World, op cit*, p285.

[13] Baroness Chalker, former Minister for Overseas Development, claimed: "Recent estimates suggest that 120million couples have limited or no access to family planning; many of them are desperate to delay the birth of their next child, or to have no more. Our task is to help meet that huge demand..." ('Children must not be a matter of chance', *Independent*, 11.7.94) Also: "...where the choice is available, women will take advantage of it." (Nafis Sadik, Executive Director of United Nations Population Fund (UNFPA), in the 1991 State of World Population Report)

[14] Kingsley Davis, 'Population Policy: Will Current Programs Succeed?' in *Population, Evolution and Birth Control*, p344.

[15] *ibid* p349

[16] *Feminism and Family Planning in Victorian England, op cit*, pp130-1.

[17] FPA   leaflet, 1971, in *This Crowded Kingdom*, p136.

[18] Kingsley Davis, 'Population Policy: Will Current Programs Succeed?' in *Population, Evolution and Birth Control, op cit*, p349

[19] Morton Williams and Hindell, in *The Fight for Family Planning*, p172.

[20] *'Problems of the Seventies: Pollution and our environment'*, Annual Conference of Labour Women, 1970.

[21] *A Birth Control Plan for Britain*, the Birth Control Campaign, 1972.

[22] *Population Concern 10-Year Review, 1991.*

[23] *Nafis Sadik, Executive Director, UNFPA, in People, Vol. 14, No. 3, 1987.*

[24] Officially, the MAP may now be bought by females aged 16 and over through pharmacies. However, in some areas girls can obtain the MAP through school nurses as part of a government scheme of 12 zones, designed to lower teenage pregnancies. The pills are available without parental knowledge or consent. (*Daily Mail*, 28.2.2001; *Daily Telegraph*, 10.10.2000)

[25] *'Give Her a Future', Population Concern Annual Report, 1985.*

[26] *ibid*

[27] *Kingsley Davis, 'Population Policy: Will Current Programs Succeed?' in Population, Evolution and Birth Control, op cit, p349.*

[28] *See Birth Control in the Modern World; also Society and Fertility.*

[29] *"The cost of abortion, keeping children in care, maintaining the deserted family, coping with juvenile and other offenders, is enormous. It must be cheaper to encourage more enlightened attitudes towards family planning." (Anna Raeburn, introduction, Advertising and Contraceptives, Birth Control Trust, 1977) Also: "It [family planning] must mean using contraception rather than being exposed to the trauma of induced abortion." (Bradman Weerakoon, Secretary-General, IPPF, in People, Vol. 14, No. 3, 1987) And: "Unfortunately, abortion continues to be the most popular form of birth control. This would not be the case if women were better educated about family planning and had access to good contraceptive services." (Dr Eva Sabatci, 'Meeting needs in Albania', in IPPF's Annual Report, 1993-4)*

[30] *Birth Control in the Modern World, op cit, p100.*

[31] *ibid*

[32] *ibid*

[33] *ibid*

[34] *ibid p101.*

[35] *See Society and Fertility; also Birth Control in the Modern World.*

[36] *Laws of Life, op cit, p123.*

[37] *Birth Control in the Modern World, op cit, p119.*

[38] *Published BIAG (Bangladesh International Action Group), 1985.*

[39] *A community of Muslims had refused to allow family planning workers to enter their village; 550 men were rounded up and taken away; of these, 180 were forcibly sterilized. ('Shah Commission of Enquiry Third and Final Report', 6.8.1978, in Robert Whelan, Choices in Childbearing: When does Family Planning Become Population Control? The Committee on Population and the Economy, 1992)*

[40] *ibid p29*

[41] *A gold chain worth 2000 rupees was given by the tea plantation growers as an incentive to be sterilized. (Sex and Destiny, op cit, pp364-5)*

[42] *ibid*

[43] 'World Hunger, Health and Refugee Problems: Summary of Special Study Mission to Asia and the Middle East', Report prepared for he Sub-committee on Refugees and Escapees, Senate Committee on the Judiciary, January 1976, p99.

[44] Gladys Cox to C. P. Blacker, 18.1.1939, SA/EUG/C75.

[45] *Sex and Destiny, op cit*, pp139-140.

[46] *Sexing the Millennium,* HarperCollins, 1993.

[47] According to the Campaign, "menstrual chaos" – heavy bleeding, continual light bleeding, or none at all – nausea, dizziness, cramps, headaches, loss of sex-drive, irritability, backache, depression, bloating and fatigue. These are called 'subjective complaints (i.e. they cannot be measured), and tend to be dismissed as unimportant.

[48] *A Report by the Campaign Against Depo-Provera*, published Black Rose, London.

[49] It was actually tried for the first time on Brazilian women in 1975 by a Professor Elsimar Coutinho, who began tests without consultation or Ministry of Health authorization, a legal requirement for human experiments. For the full story, see 'A Question of Control: Women's perspectives on the development and use of contraceptive technologies', a Report of an international conference held in Woudschoten, the Netherlands, April 1991, (Women and Pharmaceuticals Project and Health Action International, 1992)

[50] Joseph Bonnici, Ph.D., 'Safety Issues Concerning Anti-hCG Vaccines', in the *Linacre Quarterly*, August 1996. See also Judith Richter, *Vaccination Against Pregnancy: Miracle or Menace?* published BUKO Pharma-Kampagne/Health Action International, 1993.

[51] "For almost seventy years reproductive scientists have wondered whether it would be possible to immunise women against pregnancy in the way that individuals can be vaccinated against cholera or polio." (*Society and Fertility*, p141) And on p341: "It may be that vaccination against pregnancy will be perfected..." Also: "The possibility of applying immunological methods in contraception at many stages of reproduction is...now being pursued actively." (*Birth Control in the Modern World*, pp280-1) See also *Medical History of Contraception, p211*.

[52] *Vaccination Against Pregnancy: Miracle or Menace? op cit*, p11.

[53] *ibid* p5

[54] "Fear of the KB program [Indonesian national family planning] has severely undermined the efficacy of the government health system in East Timor. According to statistics in the UN World Population Report (1996), the death rate in East Timor is double that in Indonesia and the worst in Southeast Asia. Infant mortality in East Timor outstrips even that of Rwanda and Iraq. Yet women are unwilling to turn to the government health system for fear of covert injection or sterilization, nor do they trust public health initiatives that rely on injections and tablets." (Miranda Sissons, *From One Day to Another: Violations of Women's Reproductive and Sexual Rights in East Timor*, International Relations Program, Yale University, 23.6.1997)

[55] Contact: Campaign Against the Arms Trade, 11 Goodwin Street, London N4 3HQ, or tapol (The Indonesia Human Rights Campaign), 111 Northwood Road, Thornton Heath, Surrey CR7 8HW, for more details.

[56] It has been claimed that tetanus jabs given to women and girls in the Philippines were 'laced' with a long-lasting contraceptive drug which also causes miscarriage in women already pregnant. ('The Human Laboratory', *Horizon*, BBC2 TV, 6.11.95) Subsequent testing of women revealed hCG antibodies in their blood serum. Similar reports have also come from Nicaragua, Mexico and Tanzania. According to Human Life International: "allied with the World Health Organization in the development of an anti-fertility vaccine using hCG with tetanus and other carriers have been UNFPA, the UN Development Programme, the World Bank, the Population Council, the Rockefeller Foundation, the All India Institute of Medical Sciences and a number of universities, including Uppsala, Helsinki, and Ohio State." (*Catholic Times*, 14.1.96)

[57] G. Grant, *Grand Illusions: The Legacy of Planned Parenthood*, Cumberland House, Tennessee, 2000, pp.204-5.

[58] *Catholic Times*, 19.10.97.

[59] Elphis Christopher, *Sexuality and Birth Control in Social and Community Work*, Maurice Temple Smith, London, 1980, p175.

[60] Kingsley Davis, 'Population Policy: Will Current Programs Succeed?', in *Population, Evolution, and Birth Control*, p358.

[61] *Overpopulation: Everyone's Baby*, op cit, pp178-180.

[62] *ibid*

[63] George Morris MB MRCS, Secretary of the Doctors and Overpopulation Group, in evidence on the Group's behalf to the Social Services sub-committee of the House of Commons Expenditure Committee. (*Medical News*, 10.6.1976)

[64] Gallup Polls 1968, pp992, 994, 1005 and 1007.

[65] *Society and Fertility*, op cit, p87.

[66] *Population Control: Merchants and Methods*, pamphlet, Theresa Croshaw, Women for Life, 1984.

[67] A.S. Parkes, *Patterns of Sexuality and Reproduction*, OUP, 1976, p108.

[68] *Laws of Population*, op cit.

[69] *New Generation*, May 1925.

[70] Janet Chance, *The Cost of English Morals*, Noel Douglas, London, 1932, p73.

[71] Stephen Trombley, *The Right to Reproduce: A History of Coercive Sterilization*, Weidenfeld and Nicolson, 1988, p80.

[72] See *Birth Control in the Modern World*; Glanville Williams, *The Sanctity of Life and the Criminal Law*, Faber and Faber Ltd., 1958; Aleck Bourne FRCS, *A Doctor's Creed: The Memoirs of a Gynaecologist*, The Quality Book Club, London, 1962.

[73] See Clive Wood and Beryl Suitters, *The Fight for Acceptance: A History of Contraception*, Medical and Technical Publishing Co. Ltd., 1970; *The Sanctity of Life and the Criminal Law; Woman's Body, Woman's Right*; Bertrand Russell, *History of Western Philosophy*, Geo. Allen & Unwin Ltd., 1961.

[74] For more information on the catalogue of human rights abuses, see Steven W. Mosher, *A Mother's Ordeal: The Story of Chi An, One Woman's Fight Against China's One-Child Family Policy*, Little Brown, 1994; for human rights in Tibet, see Mary Craig, *Tears of Blood: A Cry for Tibet*, HarperCollins, 1992.

[75] To date, the British Labour Government, elected in May 1997 and again in 2001, has followed the example of the previous Conservative Government in their support for organisations that supply funds for birth control in China. This is a continuation of the 'united front' presented by both political parties on the issue when Labour was in opposition.

[76] "China's impressive achievements in family planning work have been widely recognised." "....whatever the level of success at present, the momentum must be kept up..." (*China's One-Child Family Policy*, Ed. Elisabeth Croll, Delia Davin, Penny Kane, Macmillan Press, 1985) "China has every reason to feel proud and pleased with its remarkable achievements in its family planning policy." (Nafis Sadik, head of the United Nations Family Planning Agency) Also: "The Chinese FPA was welcomed into the IPPF in 1991 – at the height of the forced abortion programme. *People* magazine claimed China could serve as a model for the Third World." (Fr. John Berry, *Abortion and the Triumph of Eugenics*, pamphlet, LIFE)

[77] The International Conference on Population and Development held in Cairo in 1994.

[78] *Universe*, 19.1.97

[79] "Voluntary birth control is certainly the only humane alternative to war, disease and starvation....This [Elizabeth Draper's *Birth Control in the Modern World*] is the kind of work which can help individuals, on a very personal issue, to decide for themselves before decisions are forced upon them." (Cover notes, Second Penguin Edition of *Birth Control in the Modern World*)

[80] *China's One-Child Family Policy, op cit.*

[81] *Independent,* 12.7.94

[82] *Independent, ibid*

[83] Letter, *New Statesman & Society,* 16.9.94.

[84] Bradman Weerakoon, Sec-Gen, IPPF, in 'People', Vol. 14, No.3, 1987.

[85] A.S. Parkes, *Patterns of Sexuality and Reproduction,* OUP, 1976, p109.

[86] *Too Many People,* Calder Publications. (*Independent*)

[87] 'People', Vol. 14, No. 3, 1987.

[88] *Universe,* 13.3.94

[89] It was claimed that Catholic MP Edward Leigh, who has spoken about world development issues, would take "the Vatican line" in opposing greater use of contraception. (*Daily Telegraph,* 20.7.2001; *Catholic Herald,* 27.7.2001)

[90] Frank Longford, interview with Jon Snow, Channel 4 TV newsreader. (*Catholic Herald,* 3.8.2001)

[91] "T. A. McGraw could not see anything wrong in prevention." (In *Medical History of Contraception,* p299)

[92] "Large families are hurtful to others not only as being the real source of poverty and of the struggle for existence, and therefore the principle cause of premature death, but also as contributing most powerfully to produce the widespread evils of celibacy and prostitution." (George Drysdale, *The State Remedy for Poverty, by a Doctor of Medicine, author of the Elements of Social Science,* published 1904)

[93] *Guardian,* Nov. 1994.

[94] The federally funded 'Demoiselle 2 Femme' educational programme for girls in poor districts aged 14 to 18, offered workshops on beauty, hygiene, sex education, parental relationships and college placement. Field trips were taken to top restaurants and museums, and girls volunteered for community service. The idea is to widen the horizons of those who might otherwise become young single parents. Abstinence programmes have been credited with helping to lower the US national teenage birth rate, which overall has dropped by 16%. (*TVF News,* 20.2.2000, in *Family Bulletin,* Family and Youth Concern, Summer 2000)

[95] *Daily Telegraph* (6.5.98)

[96] According to the *Independent* (6.9.94), US actress Jane Fonda was present at the Cairo Conference on Population in 1994 as the UN's 'goodwill ambassador'.

[97] The *Daily Telegraph* (9.10.97) reported that Ms. Fonda was to lead a campaign against the teaching of abstinence to children, backed by Durex, the British contraceptive manufacturer. The campaign was called 'Truth for Youth'.

[98] It is known that the Pill, like the coil, can have abortifacient properties. See John Wilks, A Consumer's Guide to the Pill and Other Drugs, ALL Inc., Stafford, Virginia, USA, 1997, ISBN 0 646 29226 9.

[99] See *Sexual Chemistry: Understanding Our Hormones, The Pill and HRT, op cit.*

[100] (*Daily Telegraph magazine,* 7.10.95, in Family Bulletin, No.82, Winter 1995/6)

[101] 'Sex Under 16?', a report commissioned by the Family Education Trust, found that only 17 per cent of the 2,000 13-15-year-olds questioned were sexually active, and 90 per cent wanted to marry to feel "secure and loved". (2000)

[102] A Government sponsored web site for teenagers (or anyone who can access the Web), 'ruthingking', advertised in teen magazines, directs youngsters to the 'Lovelife' website. This contains sexually explicit material, information on how to obtain dental dams to facilitate oral sex,

and directs teenagers to the nearest STD clinic and facility for abortion, contraception and the morning-after pill, under the repeated promise of 'confidential help'. This is part of the Government initiative for reducing teenage *pregnancy.*

[103] A controlled study conducted over a number of general practices in the Trent area found that 93 per cent of teenagers who had become pregnant had consulted a health professional "at least once" in the year before conception, 50 per cent of them being prescribed oral contraception. ('Consultation patterns and provision of contraception in general practice before teenage pregnancy: case control study', Churchill, Allen *et al, BMJ* Vol.321 19-26 August 2000, pp.486-8) This correlates with work done by Planned Parenthood's Alan Guttmacher Institute, which found that the teenage contraception failure rate is the highest of any other age group.

[104] The number of under-age girls becoming pregnant in England and Wales rose significantly to 8.6 per 1,000 girls in the second quarter of 1999. Figures for under-age pregnancies had started to fall after peaking at 9.1 per 1,000 in early 1998. Slightly more than half of pregnant under-16s have an abortion. (*Daily Mail*, 13.9.2000)

[105] 'Religion, Ethnicity and Sex Education: Exploring the Issues', a Report by the Sex Education Forum and the National Children's Bureau.

[106] See Note 99.

[107] 'Jowell aims to cut teenage pregnancies', *Daily Telegraph*, 27.11.97; 'Under-16s pregnancy rate highest for 11 years', *Daily Telegraph*, 13.3.98.

[108] In response to a letter of complaint regarding the leaflet, which was displayed at chemists, the Department of Health admitted the wording might be "misconstrued", and would be changed when reprinted. (Personal correspondence, 28.2.97)

[109] A spokesman for the "Sexual Health Branch" of the Department of Health claimed: "With regards to…clinical trials of EHC [emergency hormonal contraception] on young girls, no clinical trials specific to this age group have been undertaken in the UK." (Personal communication, 23.3.2001)

[110] *ibid*

[111] Foreword to *Advertising and Contraceptives* (Suzie Hayman, Birth Control Trust, 1977), pp2-3.

[112] *Patterns of Sexuality and Reproduction, op cit*, p70.

[113] A new magazine, 'B', said to "embrace a new view of femininity" and aiming to "concentrate more on love and relationships", nevertheless included in its first issue "Confession: I Had a Threesome"; "I Sold My Sex Scandal" and a four-page look at female masturbation complete with vibrator review. ('Out with ladettes, femininity is back in a new magazine for teenagers', *Independent*, June 1997)

[114] In 1993, concerned with a possible connection between these cultural influences and the rise in teenage pregnancies and abortions, and noting the findings of a previous study by the Family and Youth Concern organisation, the Labour Life Group conducted their own survey of teenage magazines. What we found confirmed the suspicion that teenage girls were being 'introduced' to a range of sexual activities by a barrage of provocative material which implied that such activity was normal and desirable for young girls; they were then advised on the 'Problem Page' to consult abortion referral agencies (called 'advice centres') if they suspected they were pregnant. On requesting a discussion of this worrying issue with then Shadow Health Secretary, Margaret Beckett, the Labour Life Group were told that she was too busy to meet them. (Labour Life Group Report on Teenage Magazines, and private correspondence.)

[115] In 1996, Conservative MP Peter Luff called for constraints on teenage magazines' contents.

[116] The Teenage Magazines Arbitration Panel (TMAP) was launched in November 1996. It was chaired by Dr Fleur Fisher (who has been associated with the Brook Advisory Centres and was at the time on its Medical Advisory Committee), and was composed of three representatives of

teenage magazines and four non-publisher members, one of whom acted as advisor to the Health Education Authority (HEA). The HEA spent £100,000 on funding an 'Only have sex if you want to' campaign in four teenage magazines in 1996. (Information from Family and Youth Concern, whose enquiry to the HEA as to whether they would fund a 'Only smoke if you want to' campaign, received no reply.) The new Labour Health Minister, Tessa Jowell, MP, has called upon teenage magazines to present information about contraception in a way that the young would find "interesting". *(Daily Telegraph,* 27.11.97)

[117] 'Schoolgirls are left holding the virtual baby', *Daily Telegraph,* 14.5.98.

[118] 'Something for all the family', *Independent,* 3.4.97.

[119] Interview, GMTV, 1.3.2000.

[120] For example: The children's charity Dr Barnados joined with the FPA, the Brook Advisory Centres and various representatives of Health Authorities, to produce a National Health Service report calling for children to be given contraceptives from age 11. (*Catholic Times,* 2.3.97); 'School-based sex advice cuts teenage pregnancies' (*Independent,* 28.4.97); 'Condoms for 9-year-olds: Parents do not need to know, says doctor', (*Daily Express,* 24.5.96); 'Lesson one: girls want to have sex', (*Independent,* 25.2.97)

[121] Figures from the Office of Population, Censuses and Surveys, HMSO, London.

[122] Parents Jenny and Tom Bacon formed a campaign for parental information when their daughter Caroline died after being prescribed the Pill without their knowledge at the age of 14. They collected a petition of over 10,000 signatures that they presented to then Prime Minister John Major in 1997. So far, nothing has been done. The address of their campaign, Parents Against Oral Contraception for Children, is: 2 Lyndhurst Grove, Allerton, Bradford, BD15 7AS.

[123] In Britain, 580,000 people are treated with a new STD every year – an increase of 21 per cent on 1981 figures – some are 'repeat' cases. (UK Communicative Disease Surveillance Centre, 3.1.92, in Dr Patrick Dixon, *The Rising Price of Love: The true cost of the sexual revolution,* Hodder and Stoughton, 1995, p72) Cervical cancer has been formally connected to the human papilloma virus (HPV), a sexually transmitted infection against which latex condoms are ineffective. The disease is known to be strongly linked with an early onset of sexual activity and multiple sexual partners. (*International Dateline,* December 1996; 'Medical Institute for Sexual Health', Vol 2 No 2); 'The bug that strikes before you know it: It's the most common sexually transmitted disease in Europe. Yet, despite being curable, chlamydia is making many women infertile. (*Independent,* 29.4.97) The Public Health Laboratory Service reveals that for under-16s, cases of chlamydia rose from 909 to 1,640 cases in 1999. <www.phls.co.uk>

[124] Home Office statistics showed that in 1986, 162 men were cautioned or found guilty of having sex with girls under 13, compared to only 94 in 1996; in 1986, there were 1,426 successful prosecutions of men who had sex with girls aged 14 and 15, compared to 576 in 1996. Department of Health figures showed that 8,000 girls attended NHS contraceptive clinics in 1971; by 1996-97, two different surveys showed the numbers had risen to 59,000 and 65,000, or one in ten girls aged 14 and 15. ('Fall in sex crime points to crisis in consent law,' *Daily Telegraph,* 24.2.98)

[125] Studies conducted in Canada, Colombia, France, Germany, Mauritius and the United States have demonstrated a 99% method effectiveness for the Sympto-Thermal and Temperature-Only NFP methods. A very large trial in India completed in 1996 (32,957 women months and 2,059 women over 21 months) had a method pregnancy rate of 0.86 per hundred women years (+/- 0.3), a 99.14% method effectiveness. (Bhargava *et al,* Field Trial of Billings Ovulation Method of natural family planning, *Contraception,* 1996; 53, 69-74) Trials of the Billings Ovulation Method in China have proved more successful than the IUD and effective for infertility too. (Shao-Zhen Quian *et al* and the Chinese BOM Collaboration Programme, *Bulletin of the Ovulatory Method Research and Reference Centre of Australia* Vol.27, No.4, pp.17-22, 2000)

[126] *Abortion, op cit,* pp60-61.

[127] *ibid*

[128] *Society and Fertility, op cit*, p122.

[129] *ibid* p123

[130] *Medical History of Contraception, op cit*, p417.

[131] In *Control of Life* (p229), he admits to erroneously giving the "mid-menstrual period" as the "safe period" in his earlier work, *Birth Control*, but goes on: "Nevertheless, and notwithstanding the times in which we live, I offer no apology to anyone who owes his or her existence to that error."

[132] See *Marie Stopes and the Sexual Revolution*, p65.

[133] "In the audience...was Dr Halliday Gibson Sutherland, a recent convert to the Roman Catholic Church." (*Marie Stopes and the Sexual Revolution*, p152); "...a physician named Halliday Sutherland...who had been a Catholic for three years when he wrote *Birth Control: A Statement of Christian Doctrine against the Neo-Malthusians* (1922)." (*The Birth Controllers*, p230); "...a Catholic physician, Halliday Sutherland..." (*The Fight for Family Planning*, p25)

[134] *Birth Control in the Modern World, op cit*, p334.

[135] *Society and Fertility, op cit.*

[136] *The Fight for Acceptance: A History of Contraception, op cit*, p119.

[137] *Marie Stopes: a biography, op cit*, p196.

[138] *Birth Control, op cit*, pp6-7.

[139] *ibid* p26

[140] *ibid* p31

[141] *ibid* pp32-3

[142] *British Medical Journal*, 23.7.1921, in *Birth Control, op cit*, pp33-4.

[143] *Birth Control, op cit*, p34.

[144] Quoted in the *Tablet*, 5.11.1921, in *Birth Control, op cit*, p34.

[145] *The Fight for Family Planning, op cit*, p24.

[146] Laetitia D. Fairfield, 'The State and Birth Control', *Medical Views on Birth Control* (ed. Marchant, 1926), p124, in *The Birth Controllers, op cit*, p247.

[147] *The Birth Controllers, op cit*, p265.

[148] H.B. Lees-Smith (Ed.), *The Encyclopaedia of the Labour Movement*, Caxton Publishing Co. Ltd., pp63-66.

[149] *ibid*, pp58-63.

[150] Her biography, given in the Encyclopaedia of the Labour Movement, states: "Laetitia Fairfield, M.D., took the degree of M.B., Ch.B., at Edinburgh University in1907, and the M.D. Edinburgh and D.P.H. London in 1912. After several years of hospital experience, joined the staff of the London County Council Public Health Department in 1911, and is now a Divisional Medical Officer. During the War was employed first with the R.A.M.C. in charge of W.A.A.C., and later became Woman Medical Director of the W.R.A.F....In 1923 was called to the Bar, at the Middle Temple. (p.xviii)

[151] 'Fifty years ago', *Catholic Times*, 11.8.96.

[152] *The Encyclopaedia of the Labour Movement*, op cit, pxx.

[153] *The Fight for Family Planning, op cit*, pp70-1.

[154] *Birth Control, op cit*, pp56-7.

[155] *ibid*, p57

[156] "Wells has hitherto remained untouched by charges of anti-Semitism…" (introduction, Michael Coren, *The Invisible Man: The Life and Liberties of H. G. Wells*, Bloomsbury, 1994.

[157] *Marie Stopes: a biography, op cit*, p207.

[158] *The Control of Parenthood*, 1920, in *The Right to Reproduce*, p80.

[159] *Radiant Motherhood*, in *Marie Stopes: a biography*, p181.

[160] See *Marie Stopes: a biography, op cit.*

[161] *The Fight for Family Planning, op cit*, pp44-45.

[162] The motto had been adopted in the early 1900s, and was briefly dropped when the society was re-named the New Generation League, and replaced by the image of a baby. However, after complaints from member Eden Paul about the "hideous, unwanted child" adorning the cover every month "in a magazine devoted to the propaganda of birth control", the picture was abandoned, and the motto once again took its place. (*Birth Control and the Population Question*, p197)

[163] Letter, 24.7.1922, from C.V. Drysdale to Cora Hodson, Secretary of the Eugenics Society. (SA/EUG/C92)

[164] "Writing quite in confidence I feel sure that our Society as a whole does not coincide with the Neo-Malthusian as a whole, and that between the extremes on the two sides there is a great divergence… I am sure that your own work and that of the middle group of eugenics is the meeting point of the two Societies and I hope very much that it will be possible for me to keep in touch with what you are doing, so that we may help each other in the navigation of the enormous unexplored expanse of which we get a glimpse." (Cora Hodson, Secretary of the Eugenics Society, to Bessie Drysdale, 19.7.1922)

[165] Drysdale, *Small Family System*, in *Birth Control and the Population Question in England 1877-1930*, p79.

[166] *Malthusian*, January 1916, in *Birth Control and the Population Question in England 1877-1930*, p80.

Chapter Five

EVERY CHILD A WANTED CHILD?

People still want children; neo-colonial birth control; abortion as family planning; eugenics and birth control; prophecies fall flat; who will stand up for the poor? beyond birth control.

Students of birth control history could be forgiven for concluding that their ancestors feared and loathed children, giving birth only out of ignorance and helplessness; that at best, they bore the burden of childrearing resigned in the knowledge that they were doing their bit for the continuance of the race.

Fortunately, oral history is a useful source of information on the attitudes and feelings of those who lived in a very different world – a world where social attitudes changed very little until about thirty or forty years ago, producing a radical transformation in the behaviour of those born since then.[1] Oral history should be explored by all those interested in social history, especially the history of women, the family and fertility control. For example, one woman in a socially mixed group interviewed in *Women Remember*, recalls that she "always enjoyed being a mother". Alice Berry Hart was born in 1896, and had experienced a difficult birth at the age of 44. Another interviewee also enjoyed motherhood: "In journal after journal, letter after letter, [Erica] details minutely every phrase of her children's development and their achievements, especially her daughter's."[2]

The overwhelming majority of interviewees in this survey had positive feelings towards children and motherhood, and this probably chimes in with the family experience of most people alive today.[3] However, younger British generations now experience a culture in which children are not simply accepted, but are planned and actively 'tried for'. Many young couples delay childbearing for economic reasons, chiefly because the woman's wage has become vital to the couple's income.[4]

Back in *Women Remember*, Alice Berry-Hart's sister Helen wanted a large family, though her husband disagreed. Falling unexpectedly pregnant at age 48, she had another son, who died. Alice comments: "She built her life on the fact that she was going to have another child".[5] Bessie Brennan, a working-class woman who didn't want a large family, nevertheless recalled the loss of two babies: "Nobody knows how you feel… Nobody knows…"

It is has been suggested that much infant death in the past was caused deliberately; that the lack of access to birth control was responsible for the rational decision to commit infanticide. Those who are fortunate enough to know something of their own family history are at least able to set such personal

135

knowledge against the cultivated impression that poor people routinely murdered their infants.

The author's maternal grandmother lost her firstborn twins, who were stillborn, also one of her next set of twins. She lost her eldest son at age fourteen, on his first day at work in a coal mine. In addition to this, the author's father lost a younger sister who died, aged two years, in the Workhouse. This personal experience is not uncommon among working-class people. It makes it all the more incredible to read remarks such as: "In a preconceptive era, celibacy and infanticide were virtually the only sure means of fertility control."[6]

Until relatively recent times, loss of children in infancy was a common fact of working-class life in Britain. Possibly mothers were more philosophical about it, as Elizabeth Roberts remarks: "Most women accepted the loss of their babies as a sad, but inevitable part of life; they nursed them devotedly but recognised that there was little they or the doctor could do in many cases. A few were distraught at the loss of a child. Mrs Gregson's [an interviewee's] mother had sixteen children and raised eleven: '...I can remember her carrying that little coffin with the baby in...She said that every baby she saw she wanted to snatch. She would have stolen anybody's baby to fill that want. She had all those, but she wouldn't spare one.'[7]

Phyllis Chessler's *Sacred Bond* draws attention to the strong maternal feelings of women who agree to have a baby for another woman, and subsequently change their minds.[8] Women who have lost children, like Mrs Gregson's mother, can be tempted to snatch another woman's infant to fill the void.

Still, Potts' and Selman's view is that "...the lowering of infant and child mortality, in the absence of any immediate offsetting control over births, imposes strains on the family as more children survive..."[9] Apparently they see the *survival* of children as more stressful for families than losing them.

Police officers, fire-fighters, ambulance and hospital personnel, whose work is to save lives, but who are accustomed by the nature of their work to loss of life, find the deaths of babies and children the most difficult to accept. Perhaps this is because the death of children sharply recalls their utter helplessness. Far from being enemies of our autonomy – the 'unwanted child' - in death, they can be seen as what they really are: innocent victims.

It is difficult to understand how birth control advocate Norman Himes can relate, in scrupulous detail, and without a shudder, Madagascan customs of infanticide for superstitious reasons.[10] He also relates "most interesting" cases of mutilation of African women for the "prevention of conception". Without passing judgement on the brutality meted out to these African women, Himes seems more interested in using their sufferings to prove that prevention of conception has been common in primitive peoples worldwide.[11]

It might come as a further surprise to students of birth control history - as it must have come as a shock to the early birth controllers - that there were many couples that actually *wanted* children. Some, evidently taking the birth controllers' 'wanted child' rhetoric seriously, approached the clinics for help

136

with infertility.[12] The birth controllers had come to believe that no one really wanted children, and that they were produced as a contribution to the Race, or out of ignorance of birth control.

In fact, the gold pin Stopes was so eager to experiment with was developed to *aid* conception – though it failed disastrously, which gave rise to the idea of using it as a method of fertility control. The same is true of the pregnancy vaccine.[13] Even while she lectured others on controlling births, Marie herself was anxious to become pregnant, and was devastated by the stillbirth of a child.[14]

Women who never married – and doubtless, many men, too – regret that they never had a family. As 'Miss X' recalls, in *Women Remember*: "I've had wonderful friends, that has been the great thing…. I suppose if I had been a person who had got married…if I'd had my own baby, that would have been my thing, because I always wanted to have children…"[15] These positive attitudes to children are not reflected in the annals of birth control, which are more interested in detailing various methods of killing children, born and unborn.

In an astonishing turnaround, the simple desire to have children is now portrayed as pure selfishness,[16] and the desire *not* to have children is portrayed as selfless.[17] Those who pursue technological routes in order to have children are exempted from this judgment, however, and assisted conception is viewed as laudable. Nevertheless, it can be inferred from the numbers seeking infertility advice that the vast majority of people do want children, but some couples, having put off having children until such time as their fertility is impaired, discover the hard way that you cannot plan a child.

When the first generation to be born after the Second World War was reaching sexual maturity, alarm bells began to ring, and prophecies began to pour forth. It was evident that people still wanted to go on having children, despite birth controllers' assurances to the contrary. The more realistic among them began to discuss coercion. Population conferences were held in Bucharest in 1974, and later in Mexico City, Cairo, and Beijing. Books written about the 'population explosion' were themselves so numerous as to constitute a problem.[18]

A debate on population was conducted in the *Times*, after a Parliamentary Early Day Motion[19] was brought which claimed that the population of the United Kingdom was "likely to increase by a third from 55 to 73 million by the end of the century". The Motion called for the Government to establish a population advisory body that could warn on population trends and advise government on "what steps should be taken to overcome [the difficulties arising from population growth] well in advance of crisis point." In a subsequent letter to the *Times*, the MPs involved used the language of threats and warnings mentioned in Chapter Four. They called for the "encouragement of voluntary methods of birth control…at an early stage in order to avoid the much more stringent steps which otherwise might well have to be taken at a later stage."

There was a flurry of letters, some calling for coercive measures to control the world's population: "To stabilize population may require policies and measures changing the nature of personal freedom as we now know it; at the least it suggests strong economic disincentives to having large families."[20] "Unless measures are taken now to mitigate the impact of greater demand upon diminishing resources, far more drastic, unpleasant and desperate measures are likely to be imposed by the end of the century, among them water rationing, food rationing, compulsory sterilization of every woman after the birth of a second or third child, restriction of accommodation, and so on..."[21] "What dismays me about people's continuing freedom to have as many children as they fancy – or as whose embryonic existence they are too feckless to prevent – is that, long before a state of alarm is reached concerning food shortage, the beauty of the countryside will have vanished..."[22]

The Government responded by setting up a population bureau as part of Overseas Development to "help build up British resources for giving aid in family planning to the less-developed countries which ask for it."[23] A few months later, the United Nations Economic and Social Council adopted a recommendation that UN development programmes "should be ready to finance projects 'designed to assist developing countries in dealing with population problems.'"[24] Shortly after, the World Bank, headed by Robert McNamara, gave its "...blessing, and its funds, to countries running birth control programmes..." It was reported that "Mr McNamara's own conviction of the absolute necessity for population control [was] a result of an intellectual conversion since joining the bank six months [previously].[25]

Neo-Colonial Birth Control

With the end of Colonialism and the spread of self-rule and democratic systems throughout the world (especially in Africa), old fears began to reassert themselves in the West. The Communist bloc was still strong; East and West, their diplomatic relations frozen in the Cold War, fought their surrogate battles in the small, poor countries of the world. Spies, assassinations and secret plots were employed by each side to destabilise the other.

Overshadowing this was the nuclear threat, which was supposed to have made conventional war obsolete and with it the large numbers of poor people needed to fight conventional battles. Nuclear weapons were so deadly that they could only be used as threats by countries that strove to assert themselves as world or regional powers.

1968 was the year of almost-revolution, as European college students protested about Western involvement in the Vietnam War. Western political, economic and military power was dramatically challenged on the streets of London, Paris and Berlin. The Post-war baby boom was at a most alarming stage of development.

Drysdale's and Sanger's old fears about democracy, and Stopes' fears about revolution, though not openly expressed after a World War had been fought against tyrannies strikingly similar to what they actually proposed, were still very much in the minds of the economically powerful. No longer able to control poor countries in the politically aware Sixties, they looked for more subtle ways to avert an uprising against a new kind of economic imperialism.

In December 1974, shortly after the first major international population conference held under UN auspices in Bucharest, several major US government agencies involved in foreign affairs submitted a detailed report on population control in developing countries. The CIA (Central Intelligence Agency), the Departments of State, Defense, and Agriculture, and the Agency for International Development, all contributed. The report was titled: "Implications of Worldwide Population Growth for US Security and Overseas Interests".

The National Security Study Memorandum which arose from this became the official guide to foreign policy, to be known as 'NSSM 200', a secret document only de-classified in 1990. Despite differences of emphasis by different Presidents, the policy is technically still in force until replaced by another document of equal importance.

The contributors to the report emphasised the United States' access to raw materials in the poorer countries. Population growth, it was feared, could lead to resentment of Western imperialism, especially in the young, to strikes, take-overs and nationalisations. Western corporate holdings might be "...expropriated or subjected to arbitrary intervention" as a consequence of "government action, labor conflicts, sabotage...civil disturbance" They acknowledged that a growing population in poor countries would be stronger, and "these types of frustrations are much less likely under conditions of slow or zero population growth."

NSSM 200 admitted that the purpose of population control was to serve US strategic, economic and military interests, at the expense of developing countries. The recommendations for reducing fertility applied to all the poor countries, but some were specially targeted: India, , Nigeria, Indonesia, the Phillipines, , Pakistan, Mexico, Thailand, Turkey, Ethiopia and Colombia.[26]

There was a problem, however. Outside offers of help with population programmes might be viewed with suspicion. The leaders of poor countries had therefore to be converted to the policy in their own interest. Such programmes would look better if they appeared to come from within the poor country itself. So the British Overseas Development department declared its intention of giving birth control help to "countries which asked for it". As no countries *had* actually asked for it, the last piece in the population control jigsaw was to get poor countries to do so.

Meanwhile, assertions of the rights of families to 'space' children, and of population control being fundamental to social and economic growth, were the mantras employed to persuade poor countries that the intentions were good. More importantly, they helped disarm criticism from Western aid agencies, and individuals concerned with human rights.

Realising the practical problems involved, i.e. that poor countries might not want such assistance, the report suggests that in cases where "US assistance is limited by the nature of political or diplomatic relations...or by the lack of strong government interest in population reduction programs (e.g. Nigeria, Ethiopia, Mexico, Brazil)" it would be wise to channel the assistance through "other donors and/or from private and international organizations".[27]

Thus a game of population pass-the-parcel was established, in which governments in democratic countries were able to indirectly support programmes that infringed the democratic rights of individuals in poor countries. When objections were raised about human rights, governments could pass the buck to the population control agencies, while continuing to give them enormous amounts of taxpayers' money for actually doing the work.

Pressure can be placed on aid agencies, as happened when an all-party group of British MPs, chaired by Richard Ottoway, called for government aid to development charities to be linked to population control, and that funding to groups which made no commitment to family planning should be cut.[28] Charities such as the Catholic Fund for Overseas Development (CAFOD), with its emphasis on the need for social and economic justice in order to achieve development, would be the obvious targets of such a policy.

The importance of using international organisations to "spearhead a multilateral effort in population" was not neglected by the authors of NSSM 200. The UNFPA was expected to play a key role in promoting the agenda of a few in order to give the impression that birth control was desired by the many. But there were problems. The authors recognised that the US government might be criticised because assistance to health programmes in the poor countries had been falling, while expenditure on population control programmes had been rising. They solved the problem by integrating these programmes, which made it harder to disentangle expenditure priorities, and at the same time allowed them to employ the rhetoric of integrated reproductive and health programmes for mothers and babies.

A 1977 annual report on the implementation of NSSM 200 emphasises the strategic importance of using "intermediaries" such as the UNFPA, the World Bank and the IPPF, since they could operate in countries where the United States was "not now acceptable". They could also be on both sides of the fence, manipulating local people to request birth control, then supplying it: "intermediaries like IPPF can act as local family planning advocates using local community leaders, a role no foreign government or international organization can hope to play".[29]

The United Nations Cairo Conference on Population and Development represented the culmination of the process defined in NSSM 200 and subsequent reports. Its Secretary General was Executive Director of the UNFPA, Nafis Sadik. Chairman of the Main Drafting Committee was President of the IPPF, Dr Fred Sai.[30] In the event, the Cairo Conference on Population failed in its aim, which was to get abortion recognised as an acceptable method of family planning. This objective was shifted to the conference at Beijing.[31]

An alliance had grown up to resist the importunities of the population controllers, consisting of poor countries, Islamic nations and the Vatican. Despite attempts to portray the Vatican influence as sinister,[32] the tide was beginning to turn. If it had not, tax payers' money from all over the world would have been devoted to introducing abortion as a fail-safe method of birth control in poor countries. However, the threat has not evaporated, and a campaign to oust the Vatican from UN status is now gathering speed.[33]

The birth control and abortion campaigns have always been interconnected – not just in theory, but also in practice. The original abortion law reform campaign was composed of birth control advocates, among them Dora Russell, Frida Laski and F. W. Stella Browne, and was supported by organisations such as the Women's Co-operative Guild.[34] From the beginning, women have been 'funnelled' into abortion via the birth control clinics, as was the case with Marie Stopes, Margaret Sanger and Dr Gladys Cox.[35] (Cox worked for the Malthusian SPBCC.)

It was possible, in the Thirties, for doctors to perform abortions on expectant mothers suffering from heart or kidney disease, or tuberculosis; this was considered adequate protection for the doctor concerned against prosecution. However, there was considerable medical disagreement on the need for abortions for health reasons, with London County Council doctor Laetitia Fairfield claiming that the LCC's policy of sending tubercular expectant mothers to sanatoria for cure was not universally practised by doctors. Abortion for TB was on the increase, and was said by her to be more "...a question of fashion".[36]

In the 1960s and 1970s, contraception was still marketed as the lesser evil to abortion, but by now many people knew from personal experience that failed contraception often led to pregnancy and sometimes to abortion. Population controllers also knew this: "Contraceptives are best viewed as mechanisms for extending the time taken to conceive. Although some individuals may be lucky, there is no way in which a society can achieve a low birth rate by the use of contraception alone."[37]

They began to hint at the necessity for comprehensive fertility control: "If most women need to terminate their fertility some significant time before the menopause, then they must have access to abortion and/or sterilisation. A family planning programme that excludes the surgical methods of fertility regulation is not a realistic programme."[38] In the 1960s and 1970s, with population hype becoming accepted as commonsense, the time was ripe to consider comprehensive fertility control, gambling on the growing acceptability of abortion in the West.

There is no longer any need to lecture people on population, because economic reality does the job much better. It also achieves the same results when governments provide comprehensive fertility control. The cost of living demands that women with children must now work.[39] Women must also work longer, because there will be fewer young people in future to pay the pensions of the old.[40] So although women have been told they would be liberated by having fewer children, or none at all, they must now work longer in paid employment to pay for their own pensions.[41]

Western women have been freed from children only to be tied to the employer. Because they have so little time for activities unconnected with family or paid work, they will be less likely to organise for their rights, as Victorian women did. They will gain equality of a sort – of morbidity and possibly also of mortality– but they will have lost the support of their children.[42] Women have been liberated from the frying pan, only to find themselves plunging towards the fire.

Eugenics and Birth Control

From the 1870s onwards - once it became obvious that the poor were having larger families than the rich - the fear of working-class sexuality grew and was exploited by the birth controllers. They maintained that the poor engaged in sexual relations with little more delicacy than animals, and that without birth control their tendency to reproduce would soon swamp the world. Marie Stopes addressed her flowery language to the middle classes, encouraging them to be positive about sex. For the poor, she emphasised the negative aspects of pregnancy and childbirth, and recommended sponges full of soap powder.

One of Stopes' correspondents, a medical officer of health named Sandilands, described the appalling ignorance of working-class patients for whom "'married love' consisted of drunken bouts of unchecked sexual passion."[43] The ignorance that worried Sandilands was, of course, the ignorance of contraceptives.

Even some who argued *against* contraception, like Florence Barrett, reinforced the images of bestial working-class men, with their lurid descriptions of "animalistic husbands who drunkenly fell upon them [vulnerable women] whenever lascivious passion dictated".[44] They reasoned that the use of contraceptives would increase the plight of women who would not have the 'threat' of pregnancy to deter their drunken husbands.[45] One fear of the birth controllers was that drunken men would not stop to use a sheath, or would fail to 'be careful'. Perhaps this was why they were so keen that poor women should be taught female methods of birth control like the pessary or Dutch cap.

Soloway observes: "Out of this jumble of middle- and upper-class assumptions about working-class behaviour, men were damned if they did and damned if they did not. In gratifying their bestial lust without fear of the consequences they were uncaring, thoughtless brutes. If, however, husbands were prudent and encouraged birth control practices, they were 'sordid and unnatural.' In either case it was simply assumed that wives were passive victims rather than willing partners in perversity."[46]

Different standards also applied in the dispensing of birth control. Dora Russell contrasted Dr Norman Haire's simple, bare clinic facilities at the Walworth Centre, with his own private Harley Street consulting rooms, "richly furnished with Chinese carpets, scarlet, black and gold lacquer cabinets, Chinese porcelain." He had a saying: "Sex for the proletarian is fourpence and find your own railings".[47]

Haire was simply echoing Francis Place who, to Carlile's objections that the practice of contraception would encourage vice, especially in women, stated bluntly that there was no chastity among the absolutely poor and not much in the ranks just higher – their living conditions rendered it nearly impossible.[48]

To calm middle-class fears that contraception would lead to vice, the Malthusians claimed that birth control would be a 'civilising force' on the poor. The Drysdales and Besant, heirs to a middle-class secularist tradition of self-help and self-education, "saw in family limitation the revitalization of self-help. It was not only the most effective cure for poverty, they insisted, but the least expensive."[49]

Besant, who refers coyly in *The Laws of Population* to the "sensual" aspects of the overcrowded conditions of the poor,[50] and apparently ignorant of their need for a family to provide security in old age, stressed the benefits of contraception to the poor: "...they look forward to an old age of comfort and of respectability instead of one of painful dependence on a grudgingly-given charity".[51]

In the 1960s, Elizabeth Draper echoed these sentiments, claiming: "Birth control is an instrument of civilization".[52] Joanna Bourke reinforces the lesson in her historical description of working-class attitudes to love and marriage, ending grimly. "Love was a bonus."[53]

The history of the poor is a blank page for all who care to scribble on it. Prejudice and a lack of working-class written sources have constructed a negative view of working class family life that has endured up to the present day. For example, the Nineties' English film 'Nil By Mouth' concentrates on the extreme violence of working-class men to their wives. It has received high praise for its 'realism'. Violence and brutishness is a reality for only a minority of working-class people, but it certainly is an enduring image.

How *did* working-class men behave in the early twentieth century? In the oral history *A Woman's Place*, a Mr Foster describes in his own words the intricacies of courtship in 1920s Lancashire: "You had walks... Sometimes, it would take you about a month, four Saturday nights and four Sunday nights, to pluck up courage to even speak to her... It would depend if she looked at you.... But they were never long lasting, you would speak to them, you would take them out, but you couldn't afford to take them to the pictures or anything like that. You couldn't buy them chocolates. If you had a few toffees you used to share them..."[54]

Last Letters Home is a collection of correspondence between parents and children, brothers and sisters, sweethearts, husbands and wives, all separated by the Second World War.[55] It contains many moving letters, especially from men in the forces – sometimes prisoners of war - to their wives and girlfriends. Here is a short extract (by no means exceptional): "My Darling Wife, to be,

"It is easy to sit here now, so quiet and peaceful and be able to write 20 pages on the whys and wherefores that make me love you more than anything in the whole world. I shall confine it to saying darling that my knowledge of women begins and ends with D--. It will always be that way. Sometimes D-- when I have the opportunity of looking at you quietly, I get a feeling that I want to go on my knees and worship you. It all starts from something deep down inside, something inexplicable. Unless you read this when you are quiet you will not take it quite as I mean it." The writer and his wife-to-be, both from the East End of London, married after a long separation.[56]

Perhaps poor men had gone through a miraculous change since the birth controllers first began to bewail their behaviour, and had become thoughtful, compassionate and faithful. Perhaps they had been 'civilised' by birth control.

But images of uncontrollable sexual urges, untouched by romance, can still be applied to far-away people whose personal lives and concerns are even more foreign to us. In the 1990s, a Population Concern advertisement featured a pair of slanted eyes in a dark skin (nothing else is visible), captioned "120 million acts of sexual intercourse will happen today." The text continues: "But many millions of women across the world do not have the family planning they want to separate their decision to have sex...from getting pregnant."[57] Are we meant to presume that the women in question had sexual intercourse unwillingly? The eyes look more sensual than distressed. The image, in conjunction with the text, is telling us that vast numbers of dark-skinned people have overwhelming sexual urges that must result in more births unless restrained by contraception.

Quality not Quantity

So we come full circle. From the beginning, the motive behind population control was quality control as well as quantity control.[58] Malthus' attitude to the poor as 'encumbrances' was mirrored by Annie Besant, who claimed that "War, infanticide, hardship, famine, disease, murder of the aged" were all "positive checks which keep down the increase of population among savage tribes."

She continues: "Men, women, and children, who would be doomed to death in the savage state, have their lives prolonged by civilisation, the sickly, whom the hardships of the savage struggle for existence would kill off, are carefully tended in hospitals; and saved by medical skill; the parents, whose thread of life would be cut short, are cherished on into prolonged old age; the feeble, who would be left to starve, are tenderly shielded from hardship, and life's road is made the smoother for the lame; the average of life is lengthened, and more and more thought is brought to bear on the causes of preventable (*sic*) disease; better drainage, better homes, better food, better clothing, all these, among the more comfortable classes, remove many of the natural checks to population."[59]

Besant's sentiments, strongly echoed in modern times, with talk of rationalisation, priorities, and the agonising ethical dilemmas posed by high-tech medical intervention, illustrate the real fear of population controllers. They regard social progress not with hope, but with fear, because it encourages the 'proliferation' of the weak.

Though they claimed to want social improvements, people like C. V. Drysdale were adamant that birth control had to come first, or it would be pointless. It would simply encourage population increase among the less fit, and so ruin the efforts of the social reformers. These arguments are still heard today in the context of aid to poorer countries whose efforts to provide services, it is claimed, are unable to keep up with increases in population despite efforts to introduce education, better housing and health care, etc.[60]

In his *Medical History of Contraception*, Norman Himes praises the American Dr Edward Bond Foote, born in 1854, who had a "strong hereditarian and eugenic point of view".[61] He describes W. A. Pusey's sentiments on the need for society to "try to stem the tendency to the peopling of the earth by the defective, the unfit and the incompetent" as "on the whole...sound and forward-looking".[62] He also lauds Margaret Sanger ("a woman of great vision, personal courage...") and her "struggle" for birth control – without, however, mentioning her eugenic sentiments.

Meanwhile, the great woman herself borrowed the ringing phrases of feminist rhetoric to preach eugenics, urging: "Women of the world arise – let us close the gates of our bodies against the diseased, the unfit, and bring to birth only the best, as we know it, which should be at least, a child with a sound body and a sound mind."[63] The publisher of Sanger's book, left-wing Rose Witcop, also invokes feminism in her introduction, but feels compelled to urge "...that for the sake of expediency, advice should be given by the Health Centres to those who were physically diseased, those who are mentally deficient and those whose health has been seriously impaired by repeated childbearing. This would most certainly help to check the spread of disease to future generations."[64]

Malthusians had been expressing fears about the dangers of adult suffrage since the end of the eighteenth century. What exercised them, and an increasing number of wealthy people (though by no means all), was that the unfit poor would be able to vote for ameliorations to their social conditions, paid for out of the pockets of the rich. This was intolerable.

In 1925, under the title 'Quality versus Quantity', Bessie Drysdale appealed: "Surely we cannot have Quantity and Quality at the same time." She goes on, chillingly: "The only Democracy worth working for is the one which is fit for the world it lives in...Birth control must be our first and foremost weapon in clearing the ground for the growth of a uniformly fine Quality population..."[65] By 1925, democracy had brought forth the Malthusians' worst nightmare: the first Labour government had been elected.

Boom goes Bust

When Halliday Sutherland and Laetitia Fairfield challenged the theory that population growth caused poverty, they were part of a chain of consciousness and independent thought stretching from William Cobbett and Karl Marx, to Germaine Greer, Julian Simon, Robert Sassone, Jacqueline Kasun, and Robert

Whelan in our own time. These people have called the population controllers' bluff, exposing their ideas as fallacious. But the ideas still retain their grip on our imagination, perhaps because fear is such a powerful motivator.

Nobody can grasp the reality of a 'billion' people. All we know is that it is an awful lot of people. With the astute aid of ever-climbing graphs against a sea of black faces, the population controllers can convey a fear, which is difficult to put into words without sounding racially prejudiced. Would a picture of Oxford Street, London, on a busy Saturday convey the same feeling? Yet who asks how many children the Oxford Street shoppers have, or are likely to have, or even *want* to have? Has the congestion in Oxford Street arisen because of people's ignorance and unmet need for contraception?

We are far more likely to associate such crowds with economic prosperity and wellbeing. People who readily believe that 'other people' need to control their numbers would be puzzled and annoyed to find those 'other people' thinking exactly the same about them. The desire for population control has more to do with fear and prejudice than science or common sense.

On close examination, population control as a cure for poverty does not make sense. Did the Malthusians and their philosophical heirs – all intelligent people - really believe their own rhetoric? Or could it be that the real idea behind population control is eugenics – to control the numbers of unfit? It must be obvious by the dawning of the Millennium that people continue to want children. The trick is to make sure that the poor do not produce more than the better off, and to do so under the impression that they are making a free, sensible choice.

Early birth controllers made the mistake of speaking too plainly when they tried to convert the poor. They succeeded only in antagonising them. They attempted, in a time of grievous economic distress, to convert the poor's democratically elected representatives in the Labour movement to the idea that it would be better to limit the numbers of the poor, than to tinker with the economic system. As history would show, they were more successful when speaking softly, than when they carried a big stick.

In the closing years of the twentieth century, it has at last been admitted that world population, under the influence of improved agricultural methods, industrialisation and prosperity, is slowing down.[66] Even more importantly – though admitted even more grudgingly - that Western nations are suffering from seriously depressed birth rates.[67] Yet who would think so, with the orchestrated hysteria over teenage births?

In 1987, Population Concern warned: "Only a disaster of appalling magnitude could now prevent the population of the world from reaching 6000 million by the end of the century."[68] Yet the world's population has reached this figure, with fewer people starving to death than in the last 20 years of the nineteenth century.[69] They go on to warn: "Africa's population is expected to increase from 583 million to over 875 million in the year 2000, at a time when per capita food production has been falling." Africa's population growth has now been halted by AIDs,[70] yet starvation has been caused by natural disasters and war. 'Population growth' has been responsible for the increase in the supply of food and health care. It has also caused the misery of war, because both are caused by people - though seldom the same people.

It is clear that the population prophets have become experts at shifting their arguments whenever they are proved wrong. For example, Paul Ehrlich predicted, in 1968, that millions would starve to death in the 1970s, despite aid; that the world would run out of food; that the United States would run out of crude oil, uranium, and other raw materials.[71] In fact, in 1870, as Greer points out, people *did* starve in India - when aid was withheld. The population then was 290,000,000 – by 1984, India was supporting 712,000,000. It was Malthus who inspired such callous treatment.[72]

As Robert Sassone points out, in his *Handbook on Population*,[73] oil companies have made substantial donations to American politicians over many years, and such 'scare stories' can have the effect of pushing up prices.

The positive outcomes for society it was predicted would come from a fall in the birth rate, have also been proved wrong. In 1978, Bernard Benjamin predicted that fewer children would mean better looked-after children, smaller classes in school, more nursery provision, more "intellectually-rewarding careers" for women (compared to motherhood, presumably), fewer children for adoption, less unemployment, less crime, less traffic, less crowded shopping centres, savings in public expenditure (especially maternity services) and less pressure on "our (sic) resources", national and world-wide, of space and energy. Lastly, he predicted that there would be more food "left over" to feed the hungry of the world.[74] Ironically, Benjamin's prophecies of overpopulation being associated with crime and dereliction bear far more resemblance to the Western countries' actual plight of *dwindling* birth rates.

Even while the population control bandwagon was getting under way in the 1960s, evidence was available to show that the gloomy prophets were wrong. The *Times* reported a fall in the Indian birth rate in February 1968.[75] In the same month, as thousands of children were reported starving in Nigeria and Biafra as a result of war,[76] it was also reported that world food production had, for the first time, outpaced the rise in world population.[77] July 1968 also saw further scientific confirmation that the contraceptive pill was linked to deaths caused by blood clotting.[78] Such awkward details were trampled in the rush to implement global population control.

The reason that population controllers have got it wrong so many times, is that when they write their recipes for heaven on earth, they leave out a couple of vital ingredients: politics and economics. Wealth distribution, government priorities, elections, powerful sectional interests - these are factors which shape life as we know it, and which we cannot afford to ignore. No wonder the Malthusian 'cake' has so frequently fallen flat.[79] For example, birth control literature will be scanned without success for information on unequal land distribution in poor countries.[80] A sample of figures issued by the UN in 1997 indicated that, while only 28 per cent of Haitians had access to safe water, 81 per cent had access to contraception.[81]

Perhaps one of the greatest sins of which population controllers have been guilty, is that they have distracted attention from the urgent need for social justice in the world. However, this is a guilt that we all share, as we excuse ourselves from addressing the real causes of poverty.[82]

Who will Stand up for the Poor?

Because the Churches have persisted in drawing attention to the real causes of poverty, their representatives have been attacked, both verbally and physically. Near-hysterical attacks have been launched against the Pope by some sections of the news media, for continuing to refuse to sanction artificial birth control.[83]

Meanwhile, many priests and religious throughout the world have suffered physical attack as they continue to work with the poor instead of against them. In 1996, and the beginning of 1997, at least 46 Catholic missionaries were killed, including three bishops, 18 priests, eight male religious, 13 nuns and four others.[84] In October 2000, four Italian missionary nuns were killed in Burundi.[85] This death toll is just a tiny fraction of reality. There have been rapes, death threats, kidnaps, and some individuals missing, feared dead. Why is so little media attention focussed on these deaths? Could it be that, by some, the Church is seen as strong – as an aggressor, rather than a victim?

Religion, as we have noted, has historically been seen as an obstacle to population control. Many of the early birth controllers were humanists or rationalists. As Peter Fryer points out, all leading birth controllers (excepting Stopes, who claimed to have received divine revelations concerning birth control)[86] were "convinced freethinkers".[87] He describes the birth control movement in the nineteenth century as "part of a vigorous challenge to christianity and christian notions of sin".[88] It was the printing presses of the freethinkers and secularists that kept alive the birth control ideas of Owen and Knowlton.[89]

Place, Carlile, Knowlton, J.S. Mill, Allbutt, Bradlaugh and Besant preached humanism and birth control, while the Drysdales saw birth control and humanism as inextricably intertwined.[90]

Stella Browne was militantly anti-religion.[91] Bertie and Dora Russell were humanists.[92] Ernest Thurtle, the Labour MP who introduced his ill-fated birth control Bill into Parliament in 1926, was also active in the National Secular Society and the Rationalist Press Association.[93]

Janet Chance, who claimed that most social problems stemmed from the "pernicious moral dictatorship" of those who refused to discuss sexual matters with children, reserved her bitterest attacks for the Church. In her book *The Cost of English Morals*, published in 1932, she accuses religious believers who "use compulsion; they even deny knowledge. They are the true successors of the fanatics who lit the human bonfires, and they are only the less pitiless because they do not, they could not, watch their own rack and thumbscrew". She goes on: "The priest, defeated as an incendiarist of his fellow-men, is now politically and socially putting his hand over the mouths of the doctors, the scientists and the humanitarians."

Chance predicts the gradual acceptance of the idea of fertility control – in some cases, compulsory – with chilling accuracy: "Years of research and expenditure, whether voluntary or State-aided, will gradually make contraception (and, when medically advised, abortion) practicable, acceptable, and as successful as any other human effort for the intelligent citizen and control of procreation *possibly compulsory for the degenerate, when we know who they are.* [My italics] During this long process, the Churches, unless they revise their methods, will first protest in the name of spiritual values; will then acquiesce in silence; will then restate Christianity; and finally become so coloured by the views of the more rational elements in the country that they will entirely forget their former arrogant opinions. They will have them (*sic*) presumably found some fresh embodiment for their divinely ordered tyranny."[94]

There is plenty of evidence to show that the connection between birth control and humanism has persisted to modern times. In 1996, *Humanist News* appealed for a humanist to represent them within the Pro-Choice Alliance, to continue the representation of "many years" on that body.[95] Polly Toynbee and Suzanne Moore, both influential and outspoken advocates of fertility control, are also listed as "distinguished supporters" of the British Humanist Association.[96]

Humanists have campaigned against religious schools, religious assemblies in schools, and even publicly funded chaplains in prisons, hospitals and the armed forces.[97]

Even though the religious opposition to birth control which still remains, has no practical power to prevent its spread or use, the mere refusal to see birth control as the solution to the problems of women and the poor, is enough to excite condemnation. For example, in reviewing Pope John Paul II's book *Crossing the Threshold of Hope*, Connor Cruise O'Brien bitterly attacked the Pope's stance on birth control - without, however, declaring his own affiliations[98] as Vice-President of the British Humanist Association, and Vice-President of Population Concern.[99]

In the Western world, where widespread hunger is no longer a problem, it is clear that a falling birth rate carries with it, not the solution to our problems, but an exacerbation of them. Far from wanting to kill each other as we struggle for *lebensraum,* like the cages of laboratory rats often cited by population controllers, one of the biggest problems of modern Western existence is loneliness.[100] Economic problems, played down at present, will loom large as those expecting comfortable pensions may be disappointed and shocked to find their pensions slashed – even in Japan.[101]

Once the myths of world hunger were exploded (and anyway drew too much attention to inequities of distribution), population controllers moved on to the 'environment' and 'green' issues.[102] But some scrutiny of the facts revealed that the poor countries were not guilty of being the biggest consumers of the earth's natural resources. Even small-scale environmental damage caused by poor people under economic and colonial pressures is not irreversible, as a thorough and detailed study in Kenya illustrated.[103] Those who sincerely cared for the ecology soon realised that poor people were dependent for their livelihood on their immediate environment, and were not likely to cause irreparable damage or to exploit it, unless under outside pressure to do so.

As it became increasingly clear that the Doomsday prophecies were not coming to pass, and that they were likely to lose the game, population controllers were already looking for somewhere else to plant the goalposts. They settled for 'reproductive health' and 'reproductive choice' for women.[104] Sadly, this is likely to distract attention from the real issues facing women. The real problems of the world — lack of peace, health care, education, clean water, human rights, etc. - will not be addressed. Once again, people's problems will become ammunition in the battle against people, who are seen as the real problem.

Images of poor, black people are used interchangeably to exploit whatever angle will produce most results. In Population Concern's Annual Report of 1984, we see a picture of an "elderly woman with child in urban Columbia". Three years later, and the same woman is a "battered wife waiting at a family planning clinic in Bogota".[105] One wonders what the woman in question would have made of all this. Did she know her image would be used to 'sell' birth control to gullible Westerners? Perhaps she was simply waiting for a bus. No doubt the mix-up with the photograph was a mistake, but one which reflects the historical attitude of birth controllers towards the poor.

Beyond Birth Control

In a bid to get people to accept birth control, abortion has been used as a threat and a goad of what would happen if people failed to contracept. But widespread personal knowledge of faulty birth control has made it clear that it is very often not the failure to contracept that leads to abortion, but the act of contracepting. Now even abortion advocates and contraceptive advocates admit this fact.[106]

Even while the link is being made, however, it can be glossed over. The recently launched 'Voice for Choice' campaign (with support from organisations which represent both abortion and contraception advocates), has called for easier access to abortion, while claiming that "comprehensive family planning services" will ensure that abortions will not increase. At the same time, they cite contraceptive failure as a valid reason for obtaining abortion.[107]

A curious juncture in population control history has been reached, where the two traditional arguments, far from being discarded, are now being used in tandem to boost the numbers using abortion *and* birth control. And why should not abortion be regarded as birth control, since it is being used to control births, as Laetitia Fairfield correctly realised? The change of nomenclature to 'family planning' was dictated by a wish to avoid the suggestion of population control, a desire to strike a positive note. Now that 'birth control' sounds so much more respectable than 'abortion', perhaps the time has come to bring abortion in from the cold, to shelter under the better-sounding name of its more respectable sister.

However, even while it is becoming clear that contraception does not help to avoid abortion, attempts are being made to leap frog over the argument about providing contraception to poor countries, simply by using development aid to provide them with abortion facilities.[108]

A glossy brochure *Time for Action: Reducing the dangers of pregnancy in poor societies* has been issued by the British Department of International Development. Buried within the report, under "Aims for Safer Motherhood Partnerships" is the goal: "ensure that proper abortion care and services, as defined and permitted by law and that respect women's dignity, are accessible to any woman needing them." 'MVA' (manual vacuum aspiration) is included in the variety of ways that the poor women of the world can be helped. Though apparently intended to "treat the complications of incomplete abortion", the possibilities for exploitation as a method of illegal abortion are obvious.

In the world of population control, nothing ever 'just happens'. There would be no point in proclaiming such goals if there were not already organisations ready and willing to implement them, and it is doubtful whether such goals ever emanated from Governments. It is probable that they were in fact initiated by non governmental organisations concerned with population control, and historically obsessed with the propensity of war victims to procreate uncontrollably.

Predictably, guidelines issued by the United Nations High Commission on Refugees have already recommended that refugee camps with more than 10,000 people should have both manual and electric uterine vacuum aspiration devices to "deal with the complications of unsafe spontaneous abortions". They also recommend that MVA be available where there is "legal, elective abortion".

This is part of the 'Safe Motherhood Initiative', and also includes the distribution of IUDs and post-coital fertility control. Sponsors of the SMI include the World Health Organisation, the United Nations Population Fund, the World Bank, the International Planned Parenthood Federation, and the Population Council. They are supported with funds from the Pathfinder International, and the Mellon, Ford and Rockefeller Foundations. What can only be a programme to *stop* women becoming mothers has been presented as a programme to help mothers[109] - a useful way of disarming criticism.

There has been marked reluctance on the part of Westerners concerned with development to endorse the imposition of birth control programmes on poorer countries. However, this very reluctance has been used to 'piggy-back' abortion provision to those countries instead. The British Secretary of State for

151

International Development, Clare Short, has indeed accused pro-lifers of causing "[m]uch of the demand for abortion" by refusing access to "effective contraception".[110]

In an admirable demonstration of disarming criticism of two abuses with one threat, she issued a stark warning: "Those who refuse access to effective contraception should not dare to make a fuss about abortion".[111] The use of the words "refuse access" makes it sound as though critics of population control are withholding something which people actually want.

By encouraging the concept of abortion 'services', and the idea that illegal abortion is endemic in poorer countries anyway, arguments over the advisability of birth control can be neatly circumvented, and the old rhetoric about preventing abortions by using contraception can be usefully laid aside.[112]

Thirty years ago, however, it was still plausible to suggest that more birth control could prevent abortion. Edwin Brooks, whose Private Member's Bill made contraception widely available in 1967 for social, rather than medical reasons, originally planned to introduce a Bill on abortion. When David Steel did so instead, Brooks chose family planning. Steel's Bill helped ease the passage of the family planning Bill by diverting opposition to state-funded family planning, into opposition against abortion.

But why should someone like Brooks, committed to a belief in the benefits of contraception, originally wish to sponsor a Bill on abortion? In *This Crowded Kingdom*, Brooks explains his complicated motives:

"The problem lay in arousing public concern and a political head of steam, and I thought this might be helped by a liberal Abortion Act which would for the first time reveal starkly the extent of contraceptive ignorance and sexual humiliation hitherto hidden in the unpublished backstreet statistics."[113]

Rather than start with a family planning Bill – for which, he admits, there was no public support - he opted for using the abortion issue as a goad to increase demand for contraception. He goes on to confirm this: "Later events…suggest that this is indeed happening, and that as the figures of legal abortions soar, so an increasingly anxious public opinion demands a better preventive family planning service."[114]

In the event, the Abortion Bill did help the Family Planning Bill into law. Brooks, the first President of the Conservation Society, a member of Population Countdown and the Birth Control Campaign, realised that his Bill went against the cultural grain. He blamed "Christian tradition" which had "sanctified the maternal instinct".[115] A Labour MP, Brooks recalled with satisfaction how Left-wingers turned from the issue of public ownership to 'easier' campaigns, such as free contraception.[116]

Faulty contraception has been increasingly used to validate abortion. But the old argument about needing contraception to avoid abortion is still used. The family planning organisations, once wary of spoiling their image by endorsing abortion, now join with the abortion advocacy organisations to argue for both family planning *and* abortion, each being used to justify the other.[117] Perhaps they feel that, by including abortion in the list of fertility control methods, there is the possibility that abortion can in time be seen as just another way of planning a family. In due course, as Janet Chance predicted, the idea will achieve acceptance.

Though the threat of abortion continues to be used to get women to contracept, and contraception may still be seen as preferable by abortion advocates, there can be very few family planners left who genuinely believe that contraception is necessary to avoid abortion. Why, then, bother with separate advocacy organisations at all? The answer is that although fertility control advocates accept abortion as a method of family planning, the public do not. For this reason, family planning organisations can fulfil a useful function by handing out abortifacient methods of fertility control that would not be so acceptable if they came from organisations plainly linked to abortion.

Yet this obstinate refusal to see abortion as just another method of family planning is an obstacle to population control throughout the world. If Western countries could be got to accept abortion (and abortifacients which blur the physical and psychological line between contraception and abortion), such methods would be far easier to export to the poor countries of the world.

As the decision to make MVAs and abortifacients available in refugee camps shows, it is useful to go two steps ahead of public opinion in the hope that the public will take one step in the direction you want. Perhaps it is hoped that if public opinion does not approve of aid money being devoted to abortion, they will at least not protest at aid money being devoted to contraception. And inevitably, abortion will follow. In the meantime, the refusal of religious believers and Aid Agencies to endorse contraception for the poor is used to justify making abortion available for the poor.

As Janet Chance noted after the Lambeth Conference's limited approval of contraception, "How marvellous it would have been, how real a revelation of human greatness, if the Bishops had said: "We have been wrong in this business of Birth Control, do not let us be too positive about abortion."[118] Once the religious and the Aid Agencies endorse contraception (even as the lesser evil to abortion), pressure will be applied to get them to endorse abortion.

The ultimate goal of the population controllers is to get people to accept *all* methods of fertility control, starting with the most innocuous. So we come to the fulfilment of the birth control story: abortion must be recognised by the people as just another method of controlling births. But the greatest triumph of all would be to get the people to accept that *babies* are the problem. Once this is accepted, killing will no longer be seen as undesirable, but laudable.

What population controllers fail to acknowledge (let alone protest about) is the very phenomenon, which disproves the whole population scam. For in countries such as China and India, where amniocentesis is being used to detect baby girls for abortion,[119] the natural balance between the sexes is being skewed. In India, the ratio of women to men has fallen to 93:100. In China, in the early

1990s, it was 100:117.[120] Without intervention, the ratio is about 100:105, and remains fairly constant. More boy babies are born overall, because of their relative vulnerability, though with good pregnancy care, more are now surviving.

How, then, does nature 'know' how, when and where to adjust this balance? Perhaps the simple truth is that population regulates itself. It is known that after wars, more baby boys are born.[121] Immigrants and settlers have always had large families; city-dwellers and other 'in-comers', after the first generation, tend to have smaller families.

It may be argued that if world population growth is slowing, should not the birth controllers take some of the credit? In order to answer this question accurately, it would be necessary to conduct a comparative study with a country with a similar socio-economic profile to Britain. Unfortunately, such countries have also been subjected to much the same fertility control policies. The Irish Republic might make a useful control in such an experiment; however, close proximity to the contraception and abortion available in Britain has rendered this comparison less useful. It is true that Ireland's birth rate has shadowed that of Britain at a slightly higher rate; it too is falling, but whether it will settle at the same level – 1.66 per woman – is not yet known.[122]

It is impossible to say whether the birth controllers can take credit for the drastic fall in family size in Britain. They have certainly had an effect, though some outcomes may have cancelled out others, for example, the increased use of contraceptives has meant more unplanned pregnancies for some women, but postponed fertility or acquired infertility (through sexually transmitted disease) for others. In either case, it would be difficult to argue that either group of women had been helped to plan their families.

It is likely that family size would have shrunk anyway, but in a much more ordered and less painful way than with outside interference. One unavoidable fact is that the wide dissemination of free contraceptives has encouraged many people to engage in sexual intercourse who would otherwise not have done so, and this is the most important factor in increased unplanned pregnancies and abortions. It has also been the most important factor in an explosion of sexually transmitted diseases (the vast majority of which were not common in the 1960s)[123] and consequent infertility.

Now that the unpleasant effects of an imploding population are beginning to make themselves felt, will anyone want to take credit for it? Birth control histories certainly attributed the first great drop in family size, which began in the 1870s in Britain, to Malthusian agitation.

However, when the 1960s explosion of population control books occurred, with nearly a hundred-year perspective on history, it should have been obvious that decreasing infant mortality, the rising age of marriage, better health and welfare and greater prosperity, had all played their part. It should also have been obvious that with people living longer as a result of better conditions, there would be a temporary phase when population would increase massively, as a result of there being more people alive – the very phenomenon which ushered in the Chinese population control programme.[124] Why, then, should writers of the swinging Sixties, with such an historic perspective, wish to credit the birth control campaign with responsibility for the first great drop in population?

Could it be that, in order to control the population of poorer countries for reasons already discussed, population controllers had to emphasise the part that birth control had played in reducing family size in the West? Poor countries could not then accuse Westerners of trying to impose something that had not already been 'tried and tested' on their own populations.

However, there was still the awkward problem of sex ratios, remaining constant whatever contraceptive policy was in place, whoever used contraception and whatever method they used. How to explain them? Valerie Grant, in *Maternal Personality, Evolution and the Sex Ratio*,[125] calls on eugenic theories to explain the mystery. According to reviewer Matt Ridley, these include the supposition that women are "slightly more likely to give birth to a baby of the sex they are best suited to raising". Apparently, they "unconsciously bias the sex ratio...by selective miscarriage or some other almost unnoticed (*sic*) phenomenon". Ridley concludes: "How the body does this is another question."[126] With this 'scientific' explanation of the inexplicable, we are once again warned off further enquiry by dubious theories that sex ratios are the product of a kind of folk-eugenics, with a heavy gloss of female empowerment.

To return to the problem of female feticide, it might be thought that this horror would be enough to alert population controllers to the folly of their attempts at control, even while using the rhetoric of feminism. But why should it? After all, baby girls will grow into women, and it is women who produce more babies. Professor Alan Parkes realised this in 1976: "Given a normal sex ratio, the average production of one surviving female child per woman could result in a potentially stable population. By contrast, the average production of two surviving female children could double the population every generation... A geometric increase of this kind would obviously be catastrophic in an historically short time."[127]

Although there are occasional news items centred on female foeticide – an injustice against foetuses, against women, and against humanity - the news stories peter out, and there has been no concerted international effort to stamp out such practices. The perception of the problem as being one of 'too many people', allows such abuses to be quietly forgotten.

In the same way, the AIDs epidemic in Africa has been largely ignored. It is incredible to speak of 'overpopulation' when so many Africans are dying, but of course population controllers like Sanger were calling for a moratorium on births after the carnage of the Second World War. In response to a question from the late Bernie Grant (a black Labour MP) about population in Africa, British Development Secretary Clare Short said she did not have the information to make a "judgement about whether Africa [was] over or under-populated".

She did, however, go on to insist that the "people of Africa and elsewhere are entitled to make their own decisions about the size of their families. The people of Africa will decide for themselves what the population of Africa should be."[128] It could be that AIDs will make that decision for Africa, but once again, the goalposts have been neatly shifted from population control to human rights. In reality, the present Labour Government is pursuing the previous Conservative Government's policy on population control, providing millions of pounds of tax-payers' money for population programmes in China, where there is no 'right to choose'.

Used to shifting their arguments whenever they are losing the game, the population control priests have finally uprooted the goalposts and run away with them. But one thing is certain – they will be back.

NOTES

[1] See Hitchens, *op cit.*

[2] *Women Remember, op cit.*

[3] One of my maternal grandmother's favourite sayings was "stock's as good as money" – in other words, even if you haven't got money, you have riches in your children.

[4] One man's wage is not now enough to keep a family and pay a mortgage. This ties in neatly with the population control theory that women's work is essential in curbing the birth rate. As the average age of first-time motherhood in the UK continues to rise, the birth controllers have succeeded in 'spacing' the generations, as they once advocated 'spacing' children.

[5] *Women Remember, op cit,* p30.

[6] Diggory, Potts and Peel, *Abortion, op cit,* p518.

[7] *A Woman's Place, op cit,* p165.

[8] *Sacred Bond: The legacy of Baby M,* Virago, 1990.

[9] *Society and Fertility, op cit,* p97.

[10] Apparently, children born on certain days in one tribe were killed immediately after birth "being dropped into a jar of boiling water head down, or buried in an ant hill." (*Medical History of Contraception, p8*)

[11] *ibid,* pp10-12.

[12] "Indeed physicians' files were filled with accounts of unhappy patients seeking ways to have additional children, or even a first." (*Birth Control and the Population Question in England 1877-1930, p124*) See also Naomi Pfeffer, *The Stork and the Syringe: A Political History of Reproductive Medicine,* Polity Press, 1993, for the sad history of assisted conception.

[13] *Birth Control in the Modern World, op cit,* p281.

[14] See *Marie Stopes and the Sexual Revolution,* also *Marie Stopes: a biography.*

[15] *Women Remember, op cit,* p109.

[16] "...how do we (re)gain a proper perspective on parenting as being a three-way contract between parents, child and society, not to be entered into casually or for purely selfish, instrumental motives?" (British Organisation of Non-Parents (BON) newsletter, January 1997)

[17] "In the past, women who felt total antipathy towards becoming mothers were unable to voice their feelings and were cajoled into going through the entire process." (Ruthie Smith, a

psychotherapist at the Women's Therapy Centre, in 'The mother of all questions: In the third part of our series on the five ages of women, Fiona Malcolm discusses the biggest choice our mothers never had – yes or no to babies.' (*The Independent*, 23.9.96); "One in five women of child-bearing age wants children, the lowest figure since the 1930s", 'The parental pleasure principle: Having children will change your life, but will it be for the better?', (*Independent on Sunday*, 10.3.96); "One in five women in Britain can now expect to die without bearing a child. Shock! Horror!" 'An offence against nature? Rubbish' (Joan Smith, *Guardian Weekend*, 22.4.95)

[18] To name but a few: *Population, Evolution and Birth Control* (1964); *The population Bomb* (1968); *Overpopulation: Everybody's Baby* (1973); *This Crowded Kingdom* (1973); *Little Universe of Man* (1978).

[19] An EDM is a Parliamentary device to discover the extent of support for a given issue by seeking as many MPs' signatures as possible. They can also be employed to stimulate interest in an issue, or create publicity for a chosen cause.

[20] Letter, P.E.M. Standish, Simon Senior Research Fellow, Faculty of Economic and Social Studies, (the *Times*, 6.11.68)

[21] Letter, W.T. Stearn (the *Times*, 7.11.68)

[22] Letter, Kathleen Manning (the *Times*, 9.10.68)

[23] *The Times*, 18.5.68.

[24] *ibid*, 1.8.68.

[25] *ibid*, 4.10.68.

[26] p15 of the introduction

[27] pp127-8

[28] *Independent*, 8.3.94

[29] John Smeaton, General Secretary, Society for the Protection of Unborn Children, Memorandum on the UN's World Conference on Women in Beijing, November 1995.

[30] *ibid*

[31] *ibid*

[32] 'The Pope crusades against UN birth control' (*Independent*, 16.6.94); 'Pope adamant on birth control' (*Guardian*, 25.7.94); "Fundamentalists are spreading lies about the last-minute attempt to avert a world population explosion" ('"Holy alliance" tries to wreck birth-control conference' (*Independent*, 31.8.94)); 'Vatican and Islamic clerics made "holy pact" on abortion' (*Independent*, 8.9.94).

[33] More than 100 non-governmental organisations have asked the UN Secretary-General to withdraw the Vatican's status as permanent observer to the United Nations, in opposition to the Holy See's policy on birth control and abortion. (*Catholic Times*, 20.2.2000)

[34] *The Fight for Family Planning, op cit*, p63.

[35] Colin Francome, Abortion Freedom: A Worldwide Movement, Geo. Allen & Unwin, 1984, p62; Conference on Marie Stopes by the Galton Instititute, 26.9.1996; evidence to Birkett Enquiry on behalf of the Society for the Provision of Birth Control Clinics. (MH71-21 AC Paper 26)

[36] Evidence of the LCC to the Birkett Enquiry, 13.4.1938 (MH71-26 AC Paper 132)

[37] *Society and Fertility, op cit*, p111.

[38] *ibid* pp111-2. See also *This Crowded Kingdom*, and *Overpopulation: Everybody's Baby*, for the importance of abortion to fertility control.

[39] 'Labour market boosted by women', (*Independent*, 6.2.97); 'Work does not always pay,' Lynette Burrows, (*Catholic Times*, 27.4.97)

[40] 'Sweden's welfare meltdown has lessons for Labour: An ageing population, joblessness and low growth are forcing a left-wing government to make painful cuts,' (*Independent*, 20.12.96); "Behind this great-granny bulge lies a dip in the number of those aged between 40 and 70, who do most of the caring," (*Independent*, 30.10.96)

[41] Women born after April 6th 1955 must now work until age 65 – the same retirement age as men – under government decree. The announcement was greeted without protest.

[42] Women's longer life spans will be under threat from the effects of smoking, alcohol and work-related stress traditionally associated with a male lifestyle. ('More women are turning to drink and cigarettes', (*Daily Telegraph*, 26.3.98) This is aside from the effects of fertility-control methods such as the Pill.

[43] R. Sandilands to Stopes, 15.12.24; 19, 23.1.25, Stopes Papers, Add. MSS. 58569, in *Birth Control and the Population Question in England 1877-1930*, pp263-4.

[44] Barrett, *Conception Control*, p31, in *ibid*.

[45] See *Public Health*, October 1925; *Practitioner*, July 1923, in *ibid*.

[46] *Birth Control and the Population Question in England 1877-1930*, op cit, p272.

[47] *The Tamarisk Tree*, op cit, p210.

[48] *The Birth Controllers*, op cit, p74.

[49] *Malthusian*, May 1979, p26; Besant, *Social Aspects*, p7, in *Birth Control and the Population Question in England 1877-1930*, op cit, p77.

[50] *Laws of Population*, p20.

[51] *ibid* p43.

[52] *Birth Control in the Modern World*, op cit, p14.

[53] 'Body: Making love and war', in Joanna Bourke, *Working-Class Cultures in Britain 1890-1960: Gender, Class and Ethnicity*, Routledge, 1994, p60.

[54] *A Woman's Place*, op cit.

[55] During the Second World War, many men were conscripted into the forces. Unmarried women and those without children might be conscripted for War work. Three of my Father's brothers entered the Forces during the Thirties, as a means of escaping unemployment.

[56] *Last letters home*, ed. Tamasin Day-Lewis, Macmillan, 1995.

[57] *Independent*, 30.5.96.

[58] People like Robert Dale Owen and Charles Knowlton. 'Karezza' or '*coitus reservatus*', which was invented by Alice Stockham, and practised in the American Oneida Community, had a eugenic purpose. Only those couples deemed 'fit' were allowed to procreate. (See *Medical History of Contraception*, p269ff)

[59] *Laws of Population*, op cit, pp12-3.

[60] "Rapid population increase is, in many parts of the world, a main factor in creating poverty and in making it virtually impossible for poor societies to lift themselves out of their poverty, since additional resources are immediately swallowed up by additional people." (John Habgood, Archbishop of York and Vice-President of Population Concern, Annual Report, 1993.) Curiously, he goes on: "Having said that, we should not use concern about over-population as a stick with which to beat the poorer nations."

[61] *Medical History of Contraception*, op cit, p280.

[62] From 'Social Problems of Medicine', an address before the American Medical Association, Chicago, June 9th and 10th, 1924. ('Chicago: Amer. Med. Asso. Press, 1924, pp1-33) in *Medical History of Contraception*, p314.

[63] *Family Limitation*, p13.

[64] *ibid* p3.

[65] *New Generation*, May 1925.

[66] 'Disasters', BBC2TV, 20.11.97; "Many Greens still call for compulsory birth control, denigrating those who raise the issue of civil rights as fainthearts", ('Birth rate slows down', *Universe*, 24.12.95); Forecasts by the International Institute for Applied Systems Analysis in Vienna, showed world population growth to be slowing down. (*New Scientist*, 17.2.1996); 'Defeat this "myth" of the population explosion: pro-life priest's plea for world', (*Universe*, 7.7.96); 'The real global threat: population implosion: Not enough people are being born, says Matt Ridley; and last week the UN started to worry about it,' (*Sunday Telegraph*, 9.11.97).

[67] 'Number's up for the prophets of doom' (*Daily Telegraph*, 12.10.1999)

[68] 'A Growing Concern', leaflet, Population Concern, 1987.

[69] See note 67.

[70] *Daily Telegraph*, 4.6.2001.

[71] *The Population Bomb*, 1968.

[72] *Sex and Destiny, op cit*, pp401-2.

[73] 1978

[74] *The Decline in the Birthrate: towards a better quality of life*, Birth Control Trust, 1978.

[75] *The Times*, 7.2.1968.

[76] *ibid*, 2.7.1968.

[77] *ibid*, 18.7.1968

[78] "Further confirmation of the growing volume of evidence that there is some association between the use of the contraceptive pill and thrombosis is given in today's issue of the *Lancet*. Dr Vessey, of the Medical Research Council's Statistical Research Unit, and Dr Josephine Weatherall, of the General Register Office, who have studied the available evidence, conclude that there is a relationship between use of the pill and an increase in the deaths of young women from blood clotting." ('Pill linked with blood clotting: Doctors still cautious' (*Times*, 12.7.1968))

[79] See also *Overpopulation: Everybody's Baby, This Crowded Kingdom, The Little Universe of Man*.

[80] In Barbados, in 1987, the top 10% of land owners owned 95% of the land; in Peru, 93%; in Colombia, 80%; in Guatemala, 76%; in the Lebanon, 57%; in Indonesia, 48%; in Mexico, 37%; in Bangladesh, 34%. In the UK, one per cent of the population owned 52% of the land. ('Book of International Lists', 1981, in *New Internationalist*, November 1987)

[81] In Uganda, the figures were 34 per cent and 82 per cent; in Vietnam, 36 per cent and 95 per cent. (*Humanity*, New Zealand, July 2000)

[82] "Family Planning programmes are less costly than conventional development projects, and the pattern of expenditure involved is very different. At the same time we are conscious of the fact that successful programmes of this kind will yield very high economic returns." (Robert McNamara, in 1969 President of the World Bank, and former US Secretary of Defense (Mass, Bonnie, *Population Target*, Toronto, 1976, in *Depo-Provera, a Report* by the Campaign Against Depo-Provera, London); see also Frances Moore Lappe and Joseph Collins, *World Hunger: Ten Myths*, Institute for Food and Development Policy, San Francisco, 1982, and John Clark, *For Richer For Poorer*, Oxfam, Oxford, 1986.

[83] See note 30.

[84] Reported by the Vatican missionary news service, *Fides* (*Catholic Times*, 2.3.1997).

[85] *Catholic Herald*, 27.10.2000

[86] See *Birth Control and the Population Question 1877-1930, op cit.*

[87] *The Birth Controllers, op cit*, p11.

[88] *ibid*, p12.

[89] *ibid*, p107.

[90] See *The Birth Controllers*; also Susan Budd, *Varieties of Unbelief: Atheists and Agnostics in English Society 1850-1960*, Heinemann, London, 1977.

[91] In a letter to the *Freethinker* of 20.12.1931, she refers to the "troll-like inhabitants in the shadow of the Cross"; referring to Christian prohibitions against masturbation, she states: "The black shadow of the Christian superstition has perpetuated needless ignorance and suffering here." (Browne's contribution to the British Society for the Study of Sex Psychology, read out at their meeting of 14.10.1915)

[92] See the *Tamarisk Tree, op cit.*

[93] *New Statesman and Society*, 26.8.1994.

[94] Janet Chance, *The Cost of English Morals*, Noel Douglas, London, 1932.

[95] *Humanist News*, August/September 1996.

[96] Both are listed as such in *Humanist News*, August/September 1996.

[97] 'Freethinker' leaflet, 1999

[98] *Independent*, 25.11.1994. A personal complaint regarding the bias involved in presenting Dr O'Brien's views without revealing his own affiliations, was subsequently rejected by the editor.

[99] *New Humanist*, Autumn 1995. Population Concern Report, 1993; Population Concern letter, August 1994.

[100] "Without children, this particular social group has more money to spend on themselves," 'Dinkys raise flag for the good life,' (*Independent*, 5.6.96); 'Home alone trend is a nightmare for urban planners,' (*Independent*, 6.6.96); 'Single life for homeowners', (*Independent*, 9.5.97)

[101] 'Ageing population crisis forces Japan to slash pensions' (*Daily Telegraph*, 29.3.2000)

[102] "…the damage which increasing numbers of extremely poor people are forced to inflict on the environment in their struggles for existence…" ('Environment' supplement issued with *People* (the magazine of the IPPF), vol. 14, no. 3, 1987)

[103] Tiffen, Mortimore and Gichuki, *More People, less Erosion: Environmental Recovery in Kenya*, John Wiley & Sons, 1994.

[104] 'Safer motherhood', *People*, Vol.14, No. 3, 1987.

[105] *People*, 1987.

[106] "As people turn to contraception, there will be a rise, not a fall, in the abortion rate…" (Malcolm Potts, *Cambridge Evening News*, 7.2.1973)

[107] 'Voice for Choice: The Campaign to Secure Abortion on Request Throughout the UK', leaflet, 1998; according to the leaflet, Voice for Choice is administered by the Pro-Choice Alliance (11-13 Charlotte Street, London W1 – the same address as the Abortion Law Reform Association, which set it up), and its supporters include ALRA, the Family Planning Association, the Brook Advisory Centres and the Birth Control Trust.

[108] See Valerie Riches, *Sex and Social Engineering*, Family and Youth Concern, p12, for the ways in which population control organisations campaign for 'reforms' in the laws of target countries, to include abortion, sterilization and birth control; see also Robert Whelan, *Choices in Childbearing: When does family planning become population control?*, The Committee on Population & The Economy, 1992, p41, for claims that population control organisations have set up abortion clinics in Third World countries, regardless of abortion laws.

[109] Susan E. Wills, 'The "Safe Motherhood" Initiative Targets Refugee Camps', *Harmony: voices for a just future*, Vol.6 no.5, January 1998.

[110] 'Planned Parenthood Challenges', in *Catholic Herald*, 28.11.97.

[111] *ibid*

[112] "This intransigence" [the Catholic opposition to artificial contraception] "is not likely to lead to a reduction in demand for abortion." (Naim Attallah, 'In the name of the FATHERS', *Daily Telegraph magazine*, 19.10.97)

[113] *This Crowded Kingdom, op cit*, p103.

[114] *ibid*

[115] *ibid* p2.

[116] See the *Fight for Family Planning, op cit.*

[117] Abortion advocacy organisations behind the Voice for Choice Campaign are listed as the Abortion Law Reform Association; the Birth Control Trust; the British Pregnancy Advisory Service; Christians for a Free Choice; Doctors for a Woman's Choice on Abortion; Irish Abortion Solidarity Campaign; Marie Stopes International; National Abortion Campaign; Pro-Choice Forum; Scottish Abortion Campaign; Women's Health. ('Voice for Choice', leaflet, 1998)

[118] *The Cost of English Morals, op cit*, p107.

[119] "Parents are paid to have the daughters India lost; China fights the same campaign", 'The Missing Millions', *Independent on Sunday*, 3.10.97.

[120] *ibid*

[121] Potts and Selman discuss this in *Society and Fertility*, p65.

[122] David Coleman, 'Look after mothers and the birth rate will stop dwindling' (*Daily Telegraph*, 7.8.2001)

[123] In the 1960s syphilis and gonorrhoea were common. Today there are least 25 STDs and at least 8 new pathogens. (Institute of Medicine. Thomas Eng, William T. Butler (Eds.), *The Hidden Epidemic – Confronting Sexually Transmitted Disease*, Washington DC Nat. Acadmemy Press, 1997.

[124] Life expectancy in China was well below 40 years in 1949; by the 1970s, it had risen to between 55 and 60 years. (P. Kane (Ed.), *China's One-Child Family Policy*, Macmillan Press Ltd., 1985, p.125)

[125] Routledge, 1998.

[126] *Daily Telegraph*, 26.1.98.

[127] *Patterns of Sexuality and Reproduction, op cit*, p101.

[128] House of Commons debate, reported in *Human Concern*, Autumn 1997. Ms. Short has since blamed the Catholic Church of being a "burden" against Aids in Africa, because of the Church's teaching against condoms, (*Daily Telegraph*, 12.7.2000) despite the fact that a large part of Africa's population is not Catholic. However, she has also admitted that "Africa's problem is that the multinationals aren't interested in Africa." (*Daily Telegraph*, 12.12.2000)

CONCLUSION

Will the Meek Inherit the Earth?

Birth control priests and priestesses, while employing the rhetoric of compassion, have in fact trodden on religion, culture, human rights, human sensibilities and human relationships in order to reach their goal. When challenged, they have a habit of shifting the argument as they begin to lose ground. So we have gone from population control, to women's health, to eugenics, to world hunger and the environment, to women's rights – and now to children's rights. As each prophecy is disproved, and the birth controllers look in danger of losing the game, the goal posts are once again moved to fresh ground.

There are signs that this process is about to happen again. The new enemy of population control has been identified as "parental authority", and the new battle is one for children's rights.[1] This is because population controllers see adolescent fertility in poor countries, where girls marry younger, as a threat to their population plans.[2] This is why age of consent laws are being blatantly ignored by governments in Western countries, especially Britain. We have already seen how, with the help of orchestrated panic, and using the internet, television soaps and magazines, the Malthusian gospel is being spread to young Westerners that sex = good, babies = bad. If Western youngsters can be got to contracept, we will be justified in spreading this gospel to youngsters in poor countries.

Ultimately the whole project will fail, because birth control is not the answer to people's problems; rather, it serves the needs of population controllers to control people. The notion of sexual self-control is anathema to population controllers, so instead they preach *reproductive* control as a civilising influence because, as Edwin Brooks so tellingly put it: "...hell is other people."[3]

This belief is the root of birth control. Yet if population controllers truly believe that there are too many people in the world,[4] they should set out their stall openly. It would then be possible to properly evaluate their work. People could exercise their democratic right to decide whether this work is worth pursuing, and whether public funds should be devoted to it.

In the absence of such openness, we can at least evaluate the success of birth control in achieving the benefits that it was *claimed* would accrue from its widespread adoption. Malthusians originally preached their belief that couples should have families early, and small. However, this has not worked in practice, since birth control is used mainly to postpone childbearing, and since it then became obvious that couples who start families young tend to have more children,[5] birth controllers switched their tactics to *deterring* early childbearing by using economic sanctions.[6] The original emphasis was also on 'spacing' children. Ostensibly, this enabled mothers to have a rest. But economic sanctions against childbearing have tended to result in families of one child, or two children born very close together. This is far from ideal, since such children may suffer from sibling rivalry.

Moreover, since parents gain expertise in childrearing from practice, and become more adept in parenting skills with each child, the benefits of good parenting practice which come from larger families is vanishing from our culture. So are the benefits to children from sharing and cooperation experienced in large families, and the maturing influence of looking after younger siblings.

Once it became obvious that, under the influence of economic restraints, many couples were postponing parenthood, the idea of 'early and small' was jettisoned, and commentators began to sing the praises of older parents who, they claimed, were blessed with more patience and wisdom, and were more suited to bringing up children. In practice, however, parenthood became harder for couples who had attained a high level of material comfort. They tended to be *less* able to adjust to the regime of self-denial inherent in bringing up children, and were also less physically fit.

However, for birth controllers at least, later childbearing is beneficial in many respects. It helps to reduce the birthrate by spacing the *generations*. It ensures that couples would be more *economically* fit to have children. Perhaps most significantly, pregnancies in older mothers are automatically screened for disability. Thus delayed childbearing could ensure reduced quantity and increased quality.[7] (NB This is only a theory.)

Marriages would, it was promised by birth controllers, be happier, since couples practising birth control would be more relaxed and in control of their lives, once freed from the fear of random conception.[8] In reality, British divorce rates have risen alarmingly, alongside the rising use of contraception, and the acceptance of 'planned parenthood'. Once the idea became widely accepted that marriage was *not* ordained for the procreation of children – that children were, in fact, optional – the marriage bond was weakened. Children were no longer perceived as a joint responsibility, and the married relationship suffered from an increasing lack of commitment to the future. Couples with very young children now divorce, and increasing numbers of children are now born outside of a stable relationship.[9]

Birth controllers historically based their demands for state-aided birth control on a plea of women's health. But on a number of indicators, this has not paid off. Sexually transmitted diseases have rocketed.[10] Cervical cancer has become an increasing problem for younger women, and has been linked to a sexually transmitted virus.[11] Rates of breast cancer (which is associated with older age at first birth, the pill and abortion)[12] have also remained high.[13] The response of feminists to these outcomes has been, not to tackle the root causes of such problems, but to call for ever more screening. This puts the responsibility of the problem on individual women without, however, recommending reliable methods of avoidance.

Birth control has been seen as essential for women's freedom and equality, enabling them to pursue careers hitherto closed to them. Many women have indicated that they would rather spend the first few years of their children's lives at home.[14] However, paid work for women is known to be a limiting factor in fertility,[15] whereas work for men is known to encourage larger families. Population controllers have therefore emphasised the need for more women to enter the workforce, in order to control their fertility,[16] and governments have presided complacently over the loss of millions of traditionally male jobs,[17] 'Encouraging' single mothers out to paid work has been the main plank of the present Government's policy on decreasing welfare dependency for this group of women, presumably with an eye to preventing further lapses of reproductive good manners.

Any spare time left to working women is usually devoted to their immediate family, so the role of women as a force for social change and improvement has been, indirectly, fatally weakened by birth control. The freedom bestowed by birth control is the freedom from children, and the equality is the equal opportunity to pursue a male lifestyle.

The rejection of celibacy as an option for men and women, which has gone hand-in-hand with the preaching of birth control, has also undermined the value of celibacy in society. Self-restraint, patience and self-denial are no longer affirmed. The insight and wisdom gained from the celibate lifestyle, in commenting on sexual matters, is ridiculed and attacked.

Conversely, an active sexual lifestyle is commended, with most admiration reserved for those with the greatest number of sexual contacts. To be sexually experienced is seen as desirable. The new model of aggressive female sexuality - which coincidentally mirrors that of the libertarian male - has led to a decline in women's moral status and influence, and even their physical safety. Sexual crime continues to rise,[18] with violence by young women an increasing problem.[19] The feminist response has been to concentrate on domestic violence, with the implication that it is solely a male problem.[20] Positive views of pregnancy are 'de-bunked' by influential women.[21] One best-selling woman author, famous for her popularisation of the idea that women can 'have it all', has recently called for British women to go on a 'birth strike' for ten years because of a lack of support for mothers.[22]

Women's problems are defined by modern feminism as centring on women's dependence on their husband's income, and the lack of childcare which prevents them from achieving earnings equal to men.[23] In effect, modern feminism echoes the priorities of the birth control movement, because it sees children as the problem for women.

The birth control movement has enjoyed one huge success, however. Western society has seriously taken on board the rhetoric of the wanted child, with Britain to the fore.[24] Who, after all, could disagree with it? In practice, however, it has meant that anyone embarking on pregnancy will be doing so in a private capacity. Problems arising from bringing up children will also be a private matter. Instead of ensuring that we care *more* for children, the rhetoric of the wanted child has been a get-out clause for those who do not care. It has even influenced decisions to abort by women who fear they cannot care enough for a child on their own.

The rising age of parenthood has resulted in Western societies being geared to the material concerns of people in their twenties, because people without children have more purchasing power. In a society with increased leisure and increased spending power, a wide variety of entertainment can be purchased – television, radio, video, film, theatre, computer games - where there are few limits on what can be shown. Violence and sexual activity have become commonplace forms of visual entertainment. Any notion of self-denial or even self-restraint on the part of adults in their desire to view such material, in the interests of child protection, is considered impossible and even undesirable. Society is increasingly geared to the desires of people without children, as the BBC recently confirmed in response to a complaint about graphic sex scenes on television.[25]

Children are now seen as a minority interest. It is the parents' main task to restrain their child from causing inconvenience to the rest of society. If any problems do result – truancy, delinquency, etc. - parents will be held responsible. However, they can expect no cooperation from the authorities in preventing *society* from damaging their child; that too is seen as a private problem. Children and young people's problems continue to increase, however, as figures for premature sexual experience, sexual abuse, under-age conceptions, drug taking, homelessness, unemployment, crime and suicide confirm.[26] In 1994, there were more children in children's homes than there were people held in prison.[27]

The eugenic theory was that society would benefit by valuing children so highly that couples would not reproduce thoughtlessly, but only after careful preparation – helped, of course, by birth control. In practice, society has become more selfish, geared to the interests of the most economically powerful, because the greatest impetus to make the world a better place comes from having children.

Historically, poor mothers have supported their husbands during strikes and lockouts. They have been at the forefront of campaigns for justice, such as the mothers of the Disappeared Ones in Argentina, and Mothers for Peace in Britain. Grass-roots campaigns by mothers tend to be addressed to local causes that affect children, such as drug-pushers, dangerous paedophiles and child killers and road safety. These campaigns attract little media attention, but succeed in uniting women whose lack of a public voice makes them vulnerable to misrepresentation. Without the spur to action that having children gives, the endless volumes on children's welfare are worth little more than the paper they are written on.

Even judging by the declared aims of the population control movement, it has had a very poor success rate. This should not be too surprising. After all, the birth controllers never taught anyone how to want children, how to love and care for them. Despite this, society has accepted that they were somehow experts on child care – as if the mere act of providing someone with a mechanical device, or a pill, could prepare them for having children. Now we are left with a situation in which a minority of the world's children are materially better off, but are at the same time to a degree unwanted, while the majority of the world's children are very much wanted, but are materially poor. Can anything be done?

The very least society can do, is to stop the merry-go-round for an instant, and reflect on what has gone wrong. The population control movement is one of a number of interlocking factors that have negatively affected society. It is impossible to put back the clock. But it can at least be stopped for an instant. The birth control movement should be allowed to shout their wares in the market place alongside other specific-interest groups, and only if they can prove that they have a successful remedy to any of the problems of society, should they be granted taxpayers' money for their programmes. It seems reasonable that such public moneys should not be devoted to any solution that has manifestly failed to address the problems it was claimed it could solve, in some cases even making them worse.

However, what if the birth controllers' rhetoric were to be taken at face value? Suppose society agreed to make *every* child a wanted child? This does not mean rejecting children because society or individuals cannot or will not meet their needs. It means changing society, its priorities, and its perceptions. It would certainly involve a change of heart, but it would be worth it. And it would work.

Since the problems of the world still need to be urgently addressed, it is necessary first to identify those problems in order to decide the best way to solve them. The West needs to listen to those who are suffering in order to know what they need. Problems such as preventable disease, whole-nation debt, slave labour, unsafe drinking water, slum dwellings, poor communications, land distribution and peace, are not trivial. They will require time, resources – perhaps even a redistribution of wealth. This may discomfit a society, which has got so attached to material things that it sees their acquisition as something good and laudable, while the acquisition of many children is seen as selfish.

Society might more profitably try to develop its own agenda for the future, instead of blindly following the agenda of those who have no interest in promoting the welfare of children, or of the poor, and who only muddy the waters of international debate on what the world's priorities should be.

For even if the birth control methods being pushed were totally harmless, the poor would be damaged. Public funds which should be allocated to the elimination of poverty, should not be devoted to the elimination of the poor. Billions of pounds[28] have been poured into the population control machine; yet not a crust of bread, nor a drop of milk, has ever been put into the mouth of a poor child by the promotion of birth control.

In this country, not a job has been created (apart from, presumably, in population control organisations), nor a house, school, or hospital built, by this extravagant, non-democratic use of tax payers' money.

It is too much to hope that those responsible for such a truly dreadful campaign will ever be asked to publicly justify their philosophy. Indeed, there is every sign that an historical veil will be drawn over their blunderings. Nafis Sadik and Paul Ehrlich, two prominent personalities of the birth control movement, were recently shown on television, laughingly referring to their 'mistakes' in promoting population control. This indicates that the process has already begun.[29]

The birth control bandwagon may at last be slowing, but in its careering progress it has wrecked many lives, and it is the people who will have to pick up the pieces – the dead teenaged children; the wrecked health;[30] the infertility; the increased risks of cancer; the abortions linked to contraceptive failure. When challenged, the birth controllers will no doubt once again shift their ground, and eventually uproot the goalposts and run away with them.

We owe it to humanity and to our children to trace the true history of birth control. Their prophets of doom have filled people with despair, and their priests have preached a gospel of selfishness disguised as compassion. Having succeeded in glimpsing the real faces of these prophets and priests - systematically and progressively veiled by population control advocates in the feminist and socialist movements - we are in a better position to challenge the falsehood that ordinary people would be better off without children, and that the poor are responsible for their own poverty. Even if the worst happens, and we do not succeed, the people will still triumph in the end, because attempts to repress the poor only make them increase in number.

Or will they? Even if rumours of artificial hormones in the water supply affecting human fertility prove unfounded, there are enough toxic chemicals around to do the job just as effectively.[31] Will the meek inherit the earth after all?

NOTES

[1] "The International Planned Parenthood Federation (IPPF) issued a memo to its European Network of family planning associations (FPAs), urging them to attack the concept of 'parental authority'. It wants the FPAs to lobby 44 governments ahead of next month's review of the 1990 World Summit for Children at the United Nations, New York." ('IPPF declares global war on parents' rights', 10.8.2001)

[2] "The number of young people (aged 15-24) is expected to pass the 1,000 million mark by 1990, with most of them living in the developing world. 5% of teenagers (15-19) are having a birth every year. This rises to over 20% in some African countries. Teenage pregnancies account for 10-15% of all births worldwide. Today, in the developing world, 40% of the population are less than 15 years old." (Population Concern Annual Report 1985, p.12)

[3] *This Crowded Kingdom, op cit*, p99.

[4] "The Doctors and Over-Population Group, in its evidence to the social services sub-committee of the House of Commons Expenditure Committee, suggested that Britain's population should be reduced to about 33 million, between two-thirds and a half what it is now." ('Intelligence', newsletter No.7, International Pro-Life Information Centre, July 1976)

[5] See *Society and Fertility*, p154.

[6] "...it would be flying in the face of personal experience and common sense to deny that the cumulative effect of State support policies is to encourage birth rather than birth control." (Edwin Brooks, *This Crowded Kingdom, op cit*, p15)

[7] 'Older mums do their bit for the human race: Parenthood in later life may help us all live longer', *Independent on Sunday*, 13.7.1997. (NB The article featured three 'celebrity' older mothers.)

[8] See Janet Chance, *The Cost of English Morals*, for her advocacy of birth control to improve marriage. Chance was also, however, an advocate for easier divorce.

[9] In 1971, just over eight per cent of children were born outside of marriage. By 1991, the figure had risen to 30 per cent. (John Haskey, *Population Trends*, Spring 1993, Office of Population Censuses and Surveys, HMSO, London.)

[10] The Public Health Laboratory Service has revealed that the total number of cases of sexually transmitted diseases among those under twenty reported at clinics in England rose from 18,740 in 1995 to 24,981 in 1997. There was a rise in cases of chlamydia (linked to infertility and ectopic pregnancies) of 53% between 1995 and 1997. (*Mail on Sunday*, 28.2.1999) According to the PHLS, during the 1990s, for the first time, women overtook men regarding the incidence of STDs.

[11] According to scientific research, 99 per cent of cervical cancer cases are associated with the presence of the human papilloma virus. The virus is sexually transmitted, with claims that "most women (*sic*) have the virus at some time in their lives but shake it off naturally." Cervical cancer kills 1,200 women each year in the UK. (*Daily Telegraph*, 12.3.2000)

[12] Swedish cancer specialist Olsson states, regarding studies into the aggressive spread of breast cancer in pill takers: "...the findings... in this article should prompt additional investigations in patients who at an early age used OC [Oral Contraception] or had a miscarriage or abortion... and confirm that indeed cell proliferation is higher and tumours are more aneuploid in the early exposed patient group." (Olsson H, Ranstam MA, Baldetrop B, Ewers SB, *Cancer*, 1999, p.1289), in Wilks, *op cit*, p.61.

[13] "The majority of known risk factors relate to a woman's reproductive history, and it seems highly probable that hormones, particularly oestrogen, play an important role in the development of breast cancer. None of them is amenable to prevention, although women planning to have children should be informed of the effect of age at first birth." (The official British publication on Cancer, Series MB1 no.22 Cancer Statistics: Registrations 1989. OPCS, HMSO, London, 1994) (This is in effect a nonsense – the only way women "planning to have children" could be officially identified would be by selecting those women seeking help for infertility, in which case the advice would be inappropriate. The only way this information could be made useful to women would be to counsel those women seeking contraception or abortion, or by a wholesale programme of public information.)

[14] 'Mothers pressured to return to work,' (*Catholic Herald*, 17.12.1999); 'Mothers "prefer to be at home with children"', (*Daily Telegraph*, 5.4.2000).

[15] So is cannabis (*Daily Telegraph*, 12.12.2000), making it increasingly likely that it will be to some degree legalised in Britain in the near future. Cannabis smoking is even more carcinogenic than cigarette smoking, yet while cigarettes have been restricted in recent years on health grounds, the official attitude to cannabis has become more relaxed.

[16] "British women are more likely to have jobs than most of their European counterparts, according to new figures," 'British women more likely to work' (Statistical Office of the European Community, *Independent*, 1.2.1997)

[17] Morgan, *op cit*, p.92

[18] In 1991, 29,400 sexual offences were recorded in England & Wales; in 1999, there were 37,600. (Office of National Statistics)

[19] Home Office statistics show that in 1997, 8,600 women committed violent crimes. This is low compared with 49,600 males offenders, but double the level of the 1970s. (*Daily Telegraph*, 10.5.2001)

[20] See Erin Pizzey in Pizzey, Shackleton and Urwin, *Women or Men – Who are the Victims?* Civitas, 2000, pp.23-35, for an account of how her attempts to offer a balanced view of domestic violence was rejected by feminists. Pizzey was the pioneer of women's refuges in Britain.

[21] 'The 9 month sentence: Pregnancy is not about glowing good health – it's about swollen ankles, heartburn and a burgeoning waistline. Amanda Mitchison explains why she will never be a prisoner of her body again' (*Independent on Sunday*, 26.10.1997)

[22] "Shirley Conran, the author of *Superwoman*, yesterday urged British women to go on a baby strike or marry a Frenchman and have children abroad." ('Baby strike call by 'Superwoman', *Daily Telegraph*, 7.9.2001)

[23] Holtermann, S. and Clarke, K., *Parents' Employment Rights and Childcare*, Manchester: Equal Opportunities Commission, 1992, in Patricia Morgan, *Who Needs Parents? The Effects of Childcare and Early Education on Children in Britain and the USA*, The Institute of Economic Affairs Health & Welfare Unit, 1996.

[24] In a 1990 survey of European attitudes, only 24 per cent of Britons responded that the most important role of the family in society was bringing up and educating children. In contrast to Portugal, Greece and Spain, the majority of Britons questioned saw it in terms of personal adult fulfillment. (Norman Dennis, *Who's Celebrating What*, Christian Institute, 1995, cited in Jonathan Sacks, *op cit*, p.131.

[25] "Some 70% of all households which have a television set do not include children, and it would hardly be right to limit all those viewers to a schedule of programmes and films suitable for young children." (Personal communication, BBC Viewer and Listener Correspondence, 9.7.1993)

[26] Information from the Maranatha organisation, Liverpool.

[27] 63,000 children in care; 50,000 in prison. (A. Farmer, 'Loose Ends: Shall I be Mother?' *Labour Life Group News*, Issue No.12, Christmas 1994)

[28] British contributions to IPPF/UNFPA totalled £16.5million in 1996-7; money spent on NHS abortion and contraception totalled £216million in 1995-6. (*LIFE News*, Spring 1998)

[29] 'Disasters', BBC2TV, 20.11.1997.

[30] 'A hard pill to swallow: Women who claim they nearly died from the side-effects of the Pill are sueing doctors and manufacturers for negligence', Decca Aitkenhead, *Independent*, 1.5.95.

[31] Researchers at the Population Council's Center for Biomedical Research in New York City have found that exposure to HPTE, a metabolite of the commonly used pesticide Methoxychlor, causes declines in testosterone production and contributes to male infertility. (*Environmental Health Perspectives*, 1.9.2000 pA399) Researchers in Leeds and Dublin have discovered that ewes exposed to oestrogenic chemicals experience a speeding up of the ageing of the ovaries, ending in early menopause. Dr Helen Picton of Leeds University urged more research into the apparently lowering age of menopause in humans, given that humans and sheep react similarly to this kind of chemical exposure. (Roger Highfield, *Daily Telegraph*, 2.8.2000)

BIBLIOGRAPHY

Archival sources

Collections held at the Wellcome Institute, London:
Family Planning Association
Birth Control Campaign
Birth Control Trust

Material held at the Trades Union Congress Library, London:
Labour Party Conference Reports, 1921-1927
Drysdale, George (1904) *The State Remedy for Poverty*
Leaflets, pamphlets and newsletters: SPBCC; BCT; Population Countdown; Women's Reproductive Rights Campaign; BCC; FPA; IPPF; Co-ord Against Gillick Campaign; Brook Advisory Centres; Workers' Birth Control Group; NBCA; International Marxist Group; International Pro-Life Information Centre

Official Publications

Birth Counts, MacFarlane, A. and Mugford, M., HMSO, London
Ministry of Health Memorandum on Birth Control, 1934
Report on the Royal Commission on Population, HMSO, London, 1949
Time for Action: Reducing the dangers of pregnancy in poor societies, Dept. for International Development, Health and Population Division, 94 Victoria Street, London SW1E 5JL, 1997
A Review of the role of the IPPF in China and of the work of the CFPA, Overseas Development Administration, London, 1996
Second Report of Population Activities, Overseas Development Administration, Central Office of Information, HMSO, London, 1984

Pamphlets, Journals and Newsletters

International Action Group, 'Food, Saris and Sterilization: Population Control in, Betsy Hartmann and Hilary Standing, BIAG Ltd. (1985)
Birth Control Trust (misc.)
British Organisation of Non-Parents, *Newsletter,* 1997-9
Brook Advisory Centres (misc.)
The Campaign Against Depo-Provera, 'Depo-Provera: A Report', Black Rose, London (n.d.)
Committee on Population and the Economy, *Review* (1990-1993)

Committee on Population and the Economy, Robert Whelan, 'Choices in Childbearing: When does Family Planning become Population Control?' (1992)

The Fabian Society, 'Population and the People: A National Policy' (1945)

The Fabian Society, A. Carter, 'Too Many People?' (1962)

Family Education Trust, Valerie Riches, 'Sex & Social Engineering' (1999)

Family Planning Association, Annual Report (1992-3)

Human Life International, newsletter (1994-9)

International Planned Parenthood Federation, Annual Report, 1985, 1993-4

Joseph Rowntree Foundation with the Simon Population Trust, 'Fewer babies, longer lives', John Ermisch (1990)

Labour Abortion Rights Campaign (misc.)

Labour Party women, Labour Woman *(1920s-1930s)*

The League of National Life, *National Life,* (1929-1937)

Marie Stopes clinics (misc.)

Marie Stopes International (misc.)

The New Generation League, *New Generation* (1922, 1925, 1938)

Order of Christian Unity, Dr Margaret White, 'The Safe Sex Hoax' (1998)

Oxfam, John Clark, 'For Richer for Poorer' (1986)

Population Concern, 'Working for Change' (1981-91)

Population Concern, Annual Report, 1993, 1994

Population Concern (misc.)

The Inaugural Sir David Owen Memorial Lecture, 'The Evolution of Foreign Aid', Sir W. Arthur Lewis, President of the Caribbean Development Bank, University College, Cardiff, 1971

The Second Sir David Owen Memorial Lecture, 'Population: The World Wakes Up?', Lord Caradon, University College, Cardiff, 1973

The Third Sir David Owen Memorial Lecture, 'Reflections on Doom', Lord Ashby, University College, Cardiff, 1974

The Seventh Sir David Owen Memorial Lecture, 'The Rights of Man', Judith Hart, Minister for Overseas Development, University College, Cardiff, 1979

The Ninth Sir David Owen Memorial Lecture, 'Africa: Are We Coping?', Timothy Raison, Minister for Overseas Development, University College, Cardiff, 1984

The Tenth Sir David Owen Memorial Lecture, 'Human Numbers, Human Needs: Perspectives from the Third World', Bradman Weerakoon, Sec. Gen., International Planned Parenthood Federation, University College, Cardiff, 1986

The Eleventh Sir David Owen Memorial Lecture, 'The Problems of Fertility Regulation in Africa', Fred T. Sai, Population Division of the World Bank), University College, Cardiff, 1989`

The Thirteenth Sir David Owen Memorial Lecture, 'Rethinking Development: The Strategic Role of Population Issues', Nafis Sadik, Executive Director of the United Nations Population Fund, University College, Cardiff, 1992

Tapol (UK), A. Kohen and J. Taylor, 'An Act of Genocide: Indonesia's Invasion of East Timor', London

Newspapers and Periodicals

The Times; The Daily Telegraph; The Independent; Daily Herald; The Clarion; Labour Weekly; The New Leader; The British Medical Journal; The New England Journal of Medicine; The Lancet, The New Internationalist

Primary Sources

Besant, A. (1886) *Why I am a Socialist*, Liberty and Property Defence League
Besant, Annie (1887) *The Law of Population: Its Consequences, and Its Bearing upon Human Conduct and Morals*, Freethought Publishing Company, London
Chance, Janet (1932) *The Cost of English Morals*, Noel Douglas, London
Cobbett, William (n.d., c.1853) *A History of the Protestant Reformation in England and Ireland*, Catholic Publishing Company Ltd., London
Darwin, Charles (1871) *The Descent of Man*
Hannington, Wal (1937) *The Problem of the Distressed Areas*, Victor Gollancz Ltd., London
Hubback, Eva M. (1947) *The Population of Britain*, Pelican, Harmondsworth, Middlesex, UK
Pankhurst, Sylvia (1930) *Save the Mothers*, Alfred A. Knopf Ltd., UK
Radcliffe, Walter (1967) *Milestones in Midwifery*, John Wright & Sons Ltd., Bristol, UK
Sanger, Margaret (1924) *Family Limitation*, Rose Witcop, London
Secor Florence, Lella (1956) *Progress Report on Birth Control*, Heinemann, London
Sutherland, Halliday (1922) *Birth Control: A Statement of Christian Doctrine against the Neo-Malthusians*, Harding & More Ltd., London
Sutherland, Halliday (1936) *Laws of Life*, Sheed & Ward, London
Sutherland, Halliday (1947) *Control of Life*, Burns Oates, London
World League for Sexual Reform (1929) *Sexual Reform Congress*, London

Secondary Sources

Aitken-Swan, Jean (1977) *Fertility Control and the Medical Profession*, Croom Helm, London
Aldred, Guy (1955) *No Traitor's Gait!* Strickland Press, Glasgow
Alton, David (1997) *Life After Death*, Christian Democrat Press, Ware, Hertfordshire, UK
Banks, J.A. and Olive (1965) *Feminism and Family Planning in Victorian England*, Liverpool University Press, Liverpool, UK
Banks, Olive (1981) *Faces of Feminism*, Martin Robertson, Oxford, UK
Beekman, Daniel (1977) *The Mechanical Baby: A Popular History of the Theory and Practice of Child Raising*, Dennis Dobson, London
Bolsover, P. and Minnion, J. (eds.) (1983) *The CND Story*, Allison & Busby, London

Brooks, Edwin (1973) *This Crowded Kingdom*, Chas. Knight & Co. Ltd., London
Burridge, Trevor (1985) *Clement Attlee: A Political Biography*, Jonathan Cape, London
Carver, V. and Liddiard, P. (eds.) (1978) *An Ageing Population*, Hodder & Stoughton, O.U. Press, London and Oxford
Chesler, Phyllis (1990) *Sacred Bond: Motherhood under siege*, Virago Press Ltd., London
Christopher, Elphis (1980) *Sexuality and Birth Control in Social and Community Work*, Maurice Temple Smith Ltd., London
Clune, George (1943) *The Medieval Guild System*, Brown & Nolan Ltd.
Croll, E., Davin, D. and Kane, P. (eds.) (1985) *China's One-Child Policy*, Macmillan Press Ltd., London
Daly, Mary (1979) *Gyn/Ecology*, Women's Press Ltd., London
Danon, P. (ed.) (1995) *Tried but Untested: The aims and outcomes of sex education in schools*, Family Publications, Oxford, UK
Darlington, C.D. (1978) *The Little Universe of Man*, Geo. Allen & Unwin, London
Dickens, A.G., *The Age of Humanism and Reformation*, OU Press, Bucks, UK
Dixon, Dr Patrick (1995) *The Rising Price of Love: The True Cost of Sexual Freedom*, Hodder & Stoughton, London
Donnithorne, Audrey G. (1958) *British Rubber Manufacturing: An Economic Study of Innovations*, Gerald Duckworth & Co. Ltd., London
Donovan, C., Marshall, R. (1991) *Blessed are the Barren: the Social Policy of Planned Parenthood*, Ignatius Press, San Francisco
Dowrick, S. and Grundberg, S. (eds.) (1980) *Why Children?* Women's Press, London
Draper, Elizabeth (1965) *Birth Control in the Modern World*, Penguin, Harmondsworth, Middlesex, UK
Drogin, Elasah (1980) *Margaret Sanger: Father of Modern Society*, CUL Publications, US
Duffy, Eamon (1992) *The Stripping of the Altars: Traditional Religion in England 1400-1580*, Yale University Press, London
Eisenstein, Hester (1985) *Contemporary Feminist Thought*, Unwin Paperbacks, London
Evans, M. (1982) *The Woman Question*, Fontana, London
Fromm, Erich (1982) *The Anatomy of Human Destructiveness*, Pelican Books Ltd., Harmondsworth, Middlesex, UK
Fryer, Peter (1965) *The Birth Controllers*, Secker & Warburg, London
Gittins, Diana (1982) *Fair Sex: Family Size and Structure 1900-1939*, Hutchinson, London
Glass, D.V., and Taylor, P.A.M. (1976) *Population and Emigration*, Irish University Press, Dublin, Ireland
Gordon, Linda (1990) *Woman's Body, Woman's Right: Birth Control in America*, Penguin, Harmondsworth, Middlesex, UK

Grant, Dr Ellen (1994) *Sexual Chemistry: Understanding Our Hormones, The Pill and HRT*, Cedar, London

Greer, Germaine (1984) *Sex and Destiny: The Politics of Human Fertility*, Picador, London

Guillebaud, John (1983) *The Pill*, Oxford University Press, Oxford, UK

Hall, Ruth (1977) *Marie Stopes: A biography*, Andre Deutsch, London

Hardin, Garrett (Ed.) (1969) *Population, Evolution and Birth Control: A Collage of Controversial Ideas*, W.H. Freeman and Co., San Francisco, US

Hardyment, Christina (1984) *Dream Babies: Child Care from Locke to Spock*, OUP, Oxford, UK

Himes, Norman (1963, first published 1936) *Medical History of Contraception*, Gamut Press Inc., New York

Himmelfarb, Gertrude (1995) *The De-moralization of Society: From Victorian Virtues to Modern Values*, IEA Health and Welfare Unit, London

Hitchens, Peter (2000) *The Abolition of Britain*, Quartet Books, London

Hoffer, P.C. and Hull, N.E.H. (1984) *Murdering Mothers: Infanticide in England and New England 1558-1803*, New York University Press, London

Jones, June and Thorogood, Julia (eds.) (1986) *Yesterday's Heroes*, Sarsen Publishing, Ingatestone, Essex, UK

Kasun, Jacqueline (1988) *The War Against Population: The Economics and Ideology of World Population Control*, Ignatius Press, San Francisco

LaHaye, T, Noebel, D. (2000) *Mind Siege. The Battle for Truth in the New Millennium*, Word Publishing, Nashville, USA

Lane Hensley, Jeff (ed.) (1983) *The Zero People: Essays on Life*, Servant Books, Ann Arbor, Michigan, US

Leathard, Audrey (1980) *The Fight for Family Planning*, Macmillan, London

Lewis, Jane (ed.) (1980) *Labour and Love: Women's Experience of Home and Family 1850-1940*, Basil Blackwell, Oxford, UK

Lewis, Jane (1980) *The Politics of Motherhood*, Croom Helm, London

Lewis, Jane (1992) *Women in Britain since 1945: Women, Family, Work and the State in the Post-War Years*, Blackwell, Oxford, UK

Liljestrom, R., Noren-Bjorn, E., Schyl-Bjurman, G., Ohrn, B., Gustafsson, L.H., Lofgren, O. (1982) *Young Children in China*, Multilingual Matters Ltd., Clevedon, Avon, UK

Llewelyn Davies, Margaret (ed.) (1978) *Maternity Letters from Working Women*, Virago Ltd., London

Lyons Cross, Arthur (1917) *A History of England and Greater Britain*, The Macmillan Co., New York

MacNair, R., Krane Derr, M. and Naranjo-Huebl, L. (eds.) (1995) *Prolife Feminism Yesterday and Today,* Sulzburger & Graham Publishing Ltd., New York

Marshall, Alfred (1950) *Citizenship and Social Class*, Cambridge University Press, Cambridge, UK

Marx, Karl (1978) *Wage Labour and Capital*, Foreign Languages Press, Peking, China

McElwee, W., *History of England*, Hodder & Stoughton, London

McLaren, Angus (1978) *Birth Control in Nineteenth Century England*, Croom Helm, London

McLaren, Angus (1984) *Reproductive Rituals: The perception of fertility in England from the sixteenth century to the nineteenth century*, Methuen, London

Miedzian, Myriam (1992) *Boys will be Boys: Breaking the link between masculinity and violence*, Virago Press Ltd., London

Moore Lappe, F. and Collins, J. (1982) *World Hunger: Ten Myths*, Institute for Food and Development Policy, San Francisco, US

Morris, George (1973) *Overpopulation: Everyone's Baby,* Priory Press Ltd., UK

Oakley, Ann (1976) *Housewife*, Pelican Books, Harmondsworth, Middlesex, UK

Oakley, Ann (1982) *Subject Women*, Fontana, London

Oakley, Ann (1997) *Man and Wife: Richard and Kay Titmuss: My Parents' Early Years*, Flamingo, London

O'Brien, Mary (1981) *The Politics of Reproduction*, Routledge & Kegan Paul Ltd., London

Pankhurst, Emmeline (1979, first published 1914) *My own story*, Virago Ltd., London

Parkes, Alan S. (1976) *Patterns of Sexuality and Reproduction*, Oxford University Press, Oxford, UK

Pfeffer, Naomi (1993) *The Stork and the Syringe: A Political History of Reproductive Medicine*, Polity Press, Cambridge, UK

Phillips, A., Rakusen, J. (Eds.) (1986) *Our Bodies Ourselves: A Health Book by and for Women*, Penguin Books, Middlesex, UK

Potts, M. and Selman, P. (1979) *Society and Fertility*, Macdonald and Evans, UK

Potts, D. and Diggory, P. (1983) *Textbook of Contraceptive Practice*, Cambridge University Press, Cambs., UK

Provan, Charles D. (1989) *The Bible and Birth Control,* Zimmer Printing, Monogahela, Pennsylvania, US

Rich, Adrienne (1977) *Of Woman Born*, Virago Ltd., London

Roberts, Elizabeth (1985) *A Woman's Place: An Oral History of Working-Class Women 1890-1940*, Basil Blackwell Ltd., Oxford, UK

Rose, June (1992) *Marie Stopes and the Sexual Revolution*, Faber & Faber, London

Rowbotham, Sheila (1973) *Hidden from History: 300 years of Women's Oppression and the Fight Against It*, Pluto Press, London

Rowbotham, Sheila (1977) *A New World for Women: Stella Browne – Socialist Feminist*, Pluto Press, London

Rowbotham, Sheila and Weeks, Jeffrey (1977) *Socialism and the New Life: The Personal and Sexual Politics of Edward Carpenter and Havelock Ellis*, Pluto Press, London

Rowland, Robyn (ed.) (1984) *Women who do and women who don't join the women's movement*, Routledge & Kegan Paul Ltd., London

Russell, Bertrand (1961) *History of Western Philosophy and its Connection with Political and Social Circumstances from the Earliest Times to* the Present Day, Geo. Allen & Unwin Ltd., London

Russell, Bertrand (1976) *Marriage and Morals*, Unwin, London

Russell, Dora (1977) *The Tamarisk Tree: Vol.I My Quest for Liberty and Love*, Virago, London

Russell, Dora (1980) *The Tamarisk Tree: Vol.II My School and the Years of War*, Virago, London

Russell, Dora (1985) *The Tamarisk Tree: Vol.III Challenge and the Cold War*, Virago, London

Ryan, William (1971) *Blaming the Victim*, Orbach & Chambers Ltd., London

Sacks, Jonathan (2000) *The Politics of Hope*, Vintage, London

Scarisbrick, J.J. (1984) *The Reformation and the English People*, Basil Blackwell Ltd., Oxford, UK

Seal, Vivien (1990) *Whose Choice? Working Class Women and the Control of Fertility*, Fortress Books, London

Shapiro, Rose (1987) *Contraception: A Practical and Political Guide*, Virago, London

Sharpe, Sue (1976) *Just Like a Girl*, Pelican Books, Harmondsworth, Middlesex, UK

Smith, Anne (1989) *Women Remember: An Oral History*, Routledge, London

Snitow, Stansell and Thompson (eds.) (1983) *Powers of Desire: The Politics of Sexuality*, New Feminist Library

Soloway, Richard (1982) *Birth Control and the Population Question in England 1877-1930*, Chapell Hill University North Carolina Press, US

Stevenson, John and Cook, Chris (1979) *The Slump*, Quartet, London

Stocks, Mary (1970) *My Commonplace Book*, Peter Davies, London

Stocks, Mary (1973) *Still More Commonplace*, Peter Davies, London

Suitters, Beryl (1973) *Be Brave and Angry: Chronicles of the International Planned Parenthood Federation*, IPPF, London

Summerskill, Edith (1967) *A Woman's World*, Heinemann, London

Symons, Julian (1959) *The General Strike: A historical portrait*, The Cresset Press, London

Talbot Griffith, G. (1967) *Population Problems of the Age of Malthus*, Frank Cass & Co. Ltd., Newbury Park, Essex, UK

Tawney, R.H. (1964) *Religion and the Rise of Capitalism*, (Holland Memorial Lectures, 1922), John Murray, London

Taylor, Rosemary (1993) *In Letters of Gold: The story of Sylvia Pankhurst and the East London Federation of the Suffragettes in Bow*, Stepney Books, London

Thompson, E.P. (1977) *William Morris: Romantic to Revolutionary*, Merlin Press, London

Thompson, E.P. (1984) *The making of the English Working Class*, Pelican Books, Harmondsworth

Tiffen, Mary, Mortimore, Michael and Gichuki, Francis (1994) *More People, Less Erosion: Environmental Recovery in Kenya,* John Wiley & Sons, Chichester, Sussex, UK

Tomalin, Claire (1985) *The Life and Death of Mary Wollstonecraft,* Penguin Books, Middlesex, UK

Trombley, Stephen (1988) *The Right to Reproduce: A History of Coercive Sterilization,* Weidenfeld and Nicolson, London

Ungerson, Clare (1985) *Women and Social Policy,* Macmillan Publishers Ltd., London

Von Clausewitz, Carl, trans. M. Howard and P. Paret (1976) *On War,* Princeton University Press, US

Walker, Martin (1989) *Martin Walker's Russia,* Abacus

Walkowitz, Judith R. (1991) *Prostitution and Victorian Society: Women, class and the state,* Cambridge University Press, Cambridge, UK

Walkowitz, Judith R. (1992) *City of Dreadful Delight: Narratives of Sexual Danger in Late-Victorian London,* Virago, London

Weeks, Jeffrey (1989) *Sex, Politics and Society: The regulation of sexuality since 1800,* Longman, UK

Wilks, John B.Pharm. MPS (1997) *A Consumer's Guide to the Pill and Other Drugs,* ALL Inc., Stafford, Virginia, US

Winslow, Barbara (1996) *Sylvia Pankhurst: sexual politics and political activism,* UCL Press, London

Wollestonecraft, Mary (1985, first published 1792) *Vindication of the Rights of Woman,* Penguin, Harmondsworth, Middlesex, UK

Wood, Clive and Suitters, Beryl (1970) *The Fight for Acceptance: A History of Contraception,* Medical and Technical Publishing Co. Ltd., Aylesbury, Bucks, UK

INDEX